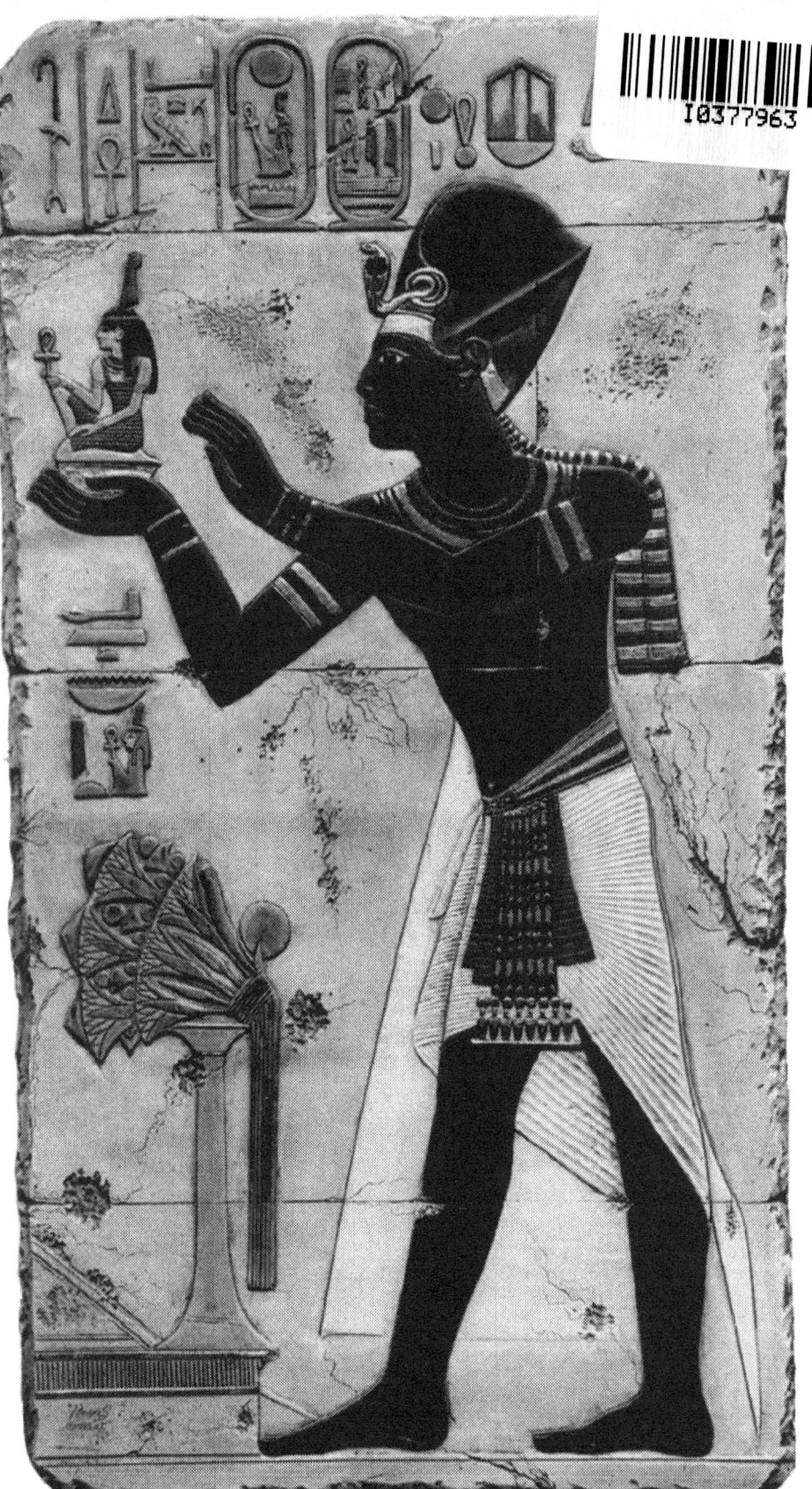

The Ancient Egyptian Wisdom Texts

Cruzian Mystic Books / Sema Institute of Yoga
P.O.Box 570459
Miami, Florida, 33257
(305) 378-6253 Fax: (305) 378-6253

© 2006 By Muata Ashby

All rights reserved. No part of this book may be used or reproduced in any manner whatsoever without written permission (address above) except in the case of brief quotations embodied in critical articles and reviews. All inquiries may be addressed to the address above.

The author is available for group lectures and individual counseling. For further information contact the publisher.

Ashby, Muata
The Ancient Egyptian Wisdom Texts: The Philosophy of Sages for Social Harmony, Metaphysical Wellbeing and Mystical Transcendence ISBN: 1-884564-65-8

Library of Congress Cataloging in Publication Data

1 Ancient Egyptian Philosophy 2 Ancient Egyptian Literature, 3 Self Help.

Also by Muata Ashby

For more listings see the back section or go online for the latest releases.

www.Egyptianyoga.com

The Ancient Egyptian Wisdom Texts

Sema
Institute of Yoga

Sema ( ) is an ancient Egyptian word and symbol meaning *union*. The Sema Institute is dedicated to the propagation of the universal teachings of spiritual evolution which relate to the union of humanity and the union of all things within the universe. It is a non-denominational organization which recognizes the unifying principles in all spiritual and religious systems of evolution throughout the world. Our primary goals are to provide the wisdom of ancient spiritual teachings in books, courses and other forms of communication. Secondly, to provide expert instruction and training in the various yogic disciplines including Ancient Egyptian Philosophy, Christian Gnosticism, Indian Philosophy and modern science. Thirdly, to promote world peace and Universal Love.

A primary focus of our tradition is to identify and acknowledge the yogic principles within all religions and to relate them to each other in order to promote their deeper understanding as well as to show the essential unity of purpose and the unity of all living beings and nature within the whole of existence.

The Institute is open to all who believe in the principles of peace, non-violence and spiritual emancipation regardless of sex, race, or creed.

Dr. Muata Abhaya Ashby

About The Author

Reginald Muata Ashby holds a Doctor of Philosophy Degree in Religion, and a Doctor of Divinity Degree in Holistic Healing. He is also a Pastoral Counselor and Teacher of Yoga Philosophy and Discipline. Dr. Ashby is an adjunct faculty member of the American Institute of Holistic Theology and an ordained Minister. Dr. Ashby has studied advanced Jnana, Bhakti and Kundalini Yogas under the guidance of Swami Jyotirmayananda, a world renowned Yoga Master. He has studied the mystical teachings of ancient Egypt for many years and is the creator of the Egyptian Yoga concept. He is also the founder of the Sema Institute, an organization dedicated to the propagation of the teachings of Yoga and mystical spirituality.

Sema Institute
P.O. Box 570459, Miami, Fla. 33257
(305) 378-6253, Fax (305) 378-6253
©1997-2006

The Ancient Egyptian Wisdom Texts

TABLE OF CONTENTS

THE FUNDAMENTAL PRINCIPLES OF ANCIENT EGYPTIAN RELIGION 6
- Summary of Ancient Egyptian Religion 16
- "The practice of the Shedy disciplines leads to knowing oneself and the Divine. This is called being True of Speech" 17
- Neterian Great Truths 18
- The Spiritual Culture and the Purpose of Life: Shetaut Neter 20
- Shetaut Neter............ 20
- Who is Neter in Kamitan Religion?.................. 21
  - The Great Awakening of Neterian Religion 22
  - Sacred Scriptures of Shetaut Neter 24

SHETAUT ASAR-ASET-HERU 24

(C. 1580 B.C.E.-ROMAN PERIOD) 24

(C. 3,000 B.C.E. – PTOLEMAIC PERIOD)............ 24
- Neter and the Neteru 25
- The Neteru 25
- The General Principles of Shetaut Neter 27
  - Medu Neter 28
  - Hekau, Medu Neter and Shetitu............ 29

ANCIENT EGYPTIAN PROVERBS ON THE PURPOSE OF LIFE AND THE VALUE OF WISDOM TEACHINGS 31

HOW TO BE A WORTHY ASPIRANT TO BE ADMITTED TO THE WISDOM TEACHINGS 34

HOW TO LISTEN, REFLECT AND MEDITATE ON THE WISDOM TEACHINGS 38
- Listening to the Teachings 38

THE SIGNIFICANCE OF THE ANCIENT EGYPTIAN WISDOM TEXTS............ 43

The Ancient Egyptian Wisdom Texts

THE TEACHINGS OF KAGEMNI 79
THE TEACHINGS OF SAGE ANI 86
THE TEACHINGS OF DUAUF 96
THE TEACHINGS OF MERIKARA 102
   Commentary by Muata Ashby 113
THE TEACHINGS OF SEHTPABRI 131
SONG OF THE HARPER 148
OTHER BOOKS FROM C M BOOKS 150

The Ancient Egyptian Wisdom Texts

Where is the land of Egypt?

A map of North East Africa showing the location of the land of *Ta-Meri* or *Kamut,* also known as Ancient Egypt.

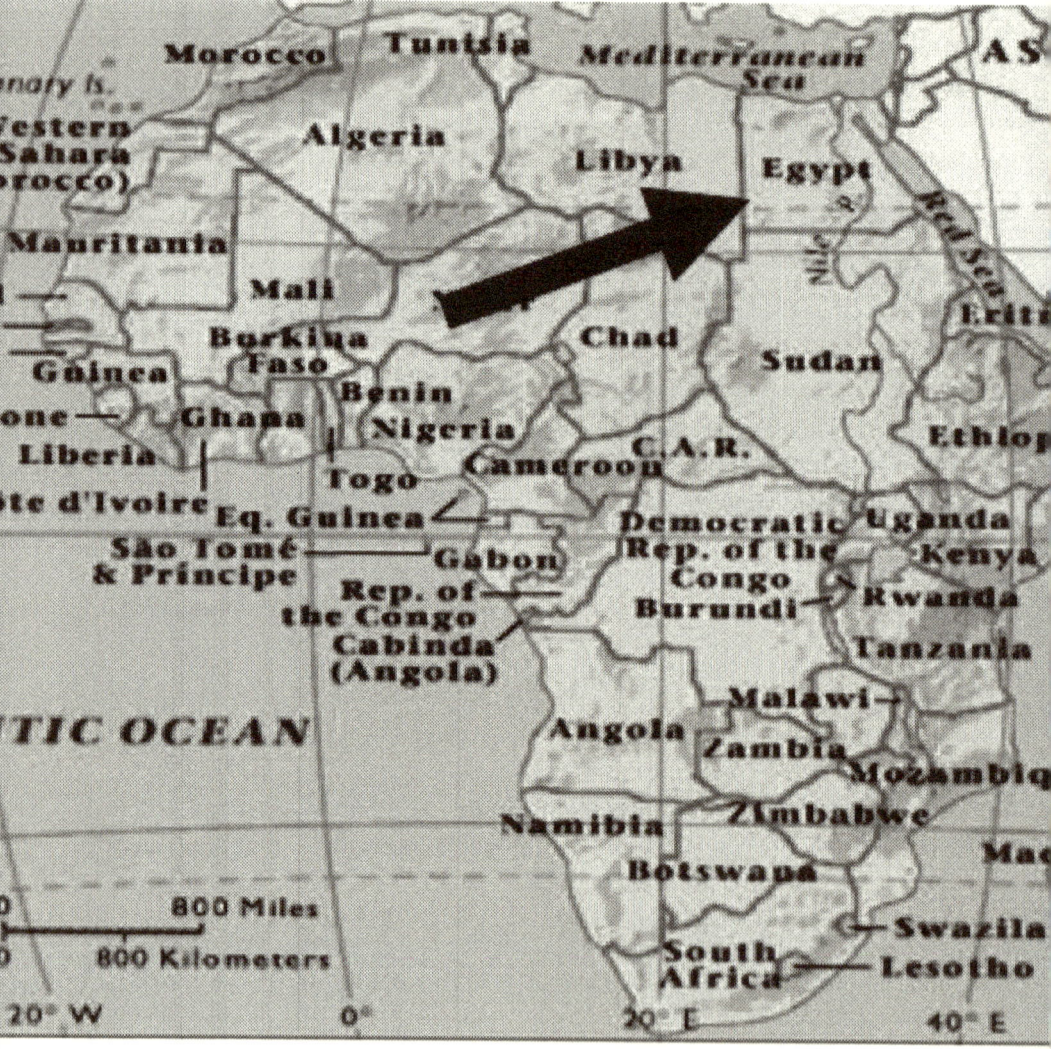

The Ancient Egyptian Wisdom Texts

The Ancient Egyptians lived for thousands of years in the northeastern corner of the African continent in the area known as the Nile Valley. The Nile River was a source of dependable enrichment for the land and allowed them to prosper for a very long time. Their prosperity was so great that they created art, culture, religion, philosophy and a civilization which has not been duplicated ever since. The Ancient Kamitans (Egyptians) based their government and business concerns on spiritual values and therefore, enjoyed an orderly society which included equality between the sexes, and a legal system based on universal spiritual laws. The *Egyptian Mystery System* is a tribute to their history, culture and legacy. As historical insights unfold, it becomes clearer that modern culture has derived its basis from Ancient Egypt, though the credit is not often given, nor the integrity of the practices maintained in the new religions. This is another important reason to study Ancient Egyptian Philosophy, to discover the principles which allowed their civilization to prosper over a period of thousands of years in order to bring our systems of government, religion and social structures to a harmony with ourselves, humanity and with nature.

The flow of the Nile brought annual floods to the Nile Valley and this provided irrigation and new soil nutrients every year that allowed for regular crops when worked on time. This regularity and balance of nature inspired the population to adopt a culture of order and duty based on cosmic order: Maat. This idea extends to the understanding of Divine justice and reciprocity. So if work is performed on time and in cooperation with nature, there will be order, balance and peace as well as prosperity in life.

Kamit (Egypt) is located in the north-eastern corner of the continent of Africa. It is composed of towns along the banks of the Hapi (Nile River). In the north there is the Nile Delta region where the river contacts the Mediterranean Sea. This part is referred to as the North or Lower Egypt, "lower," because that is the lowest elevation and the river flows from south to north. The middle of the country is referred to as Middle Egypt. The south is referred to as Upper Egypt because it is the higher elevation and the river flows from there to the north. The south is the older region of the dynastic civilization and the middle and north are later.

The Ancient Egyptian Wisdom Texts

From Ancient times Egypt was regarded by the Ancient Egyptians as being composed of three regions: Upper Egypt (south), Middle Egypt (middle), and Lower Egypt (north).

The Ancient Egyptian Wisdom Texts

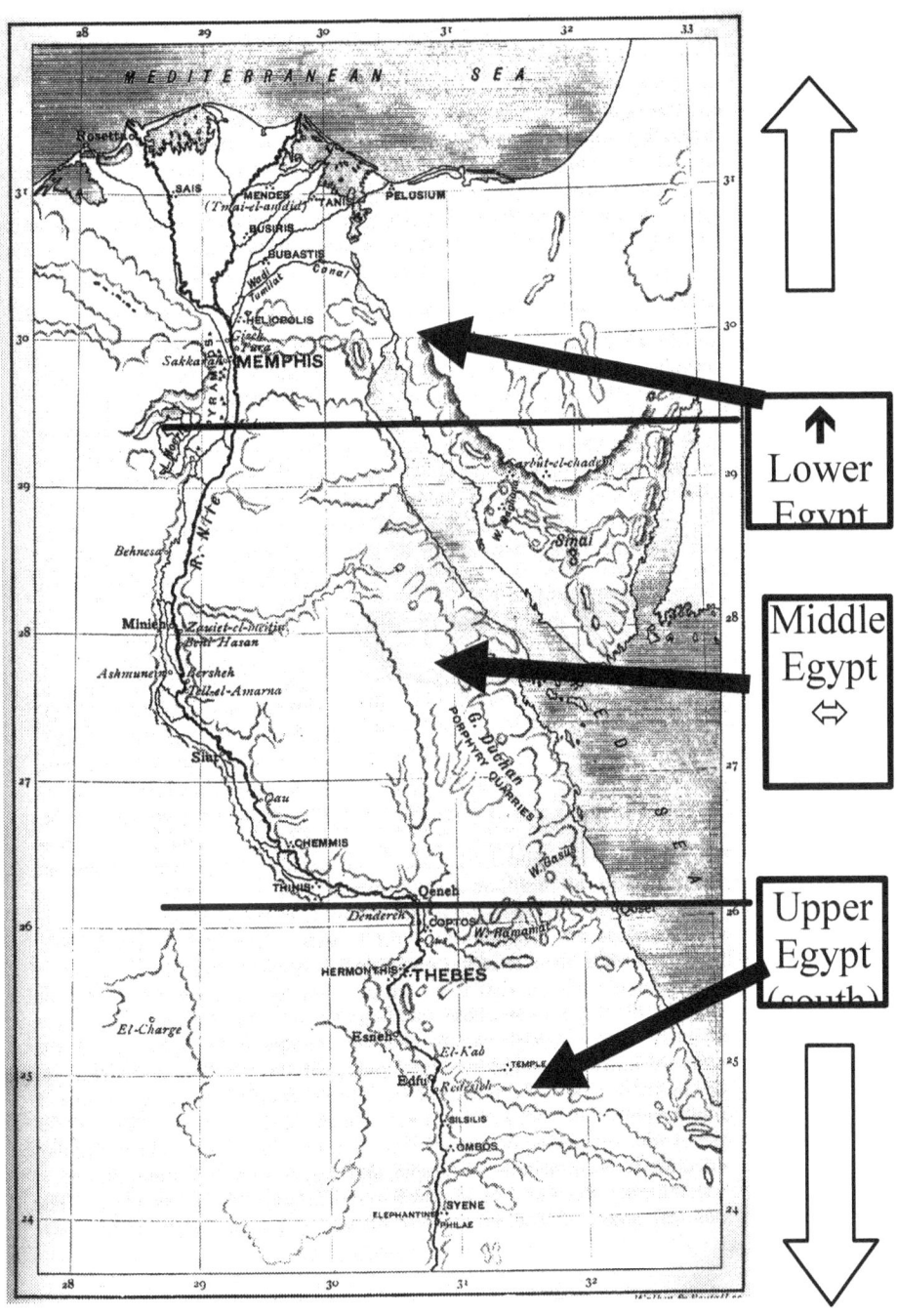

The Ancient Egyptian Wisdom Texts

Below- The Ancient Egyptian cities were related to certain divinities and their respective religious theologies. The Land of Ancient Egypt-Nile Valley - The cities wherein the theology of the Trinity of Amun-Ra-Ptah was developed were: A- Sais (temple of Net), B- Anu (Heliopolis- temple of Ra), C-Men-nefer or Hetkaptah (Memphis, temple of Ptah), and D- Sakkara (Pyramid Texts), E- Akhet-Aton (City of Akhnaton, temple of Aton), F- Abdu (temple of Asar)-Greek Abydos, G- Denderah (temple of Hetheru), H- Waset (Thebes, temple of Amun), I- Edfu (temple of Heru), J- Philae (temple of Aset). The cities wherein the theology of the Trinity of Asar-Aset-Heru was developed were Anu, Abdu, Philae, Denderah and Edfu.

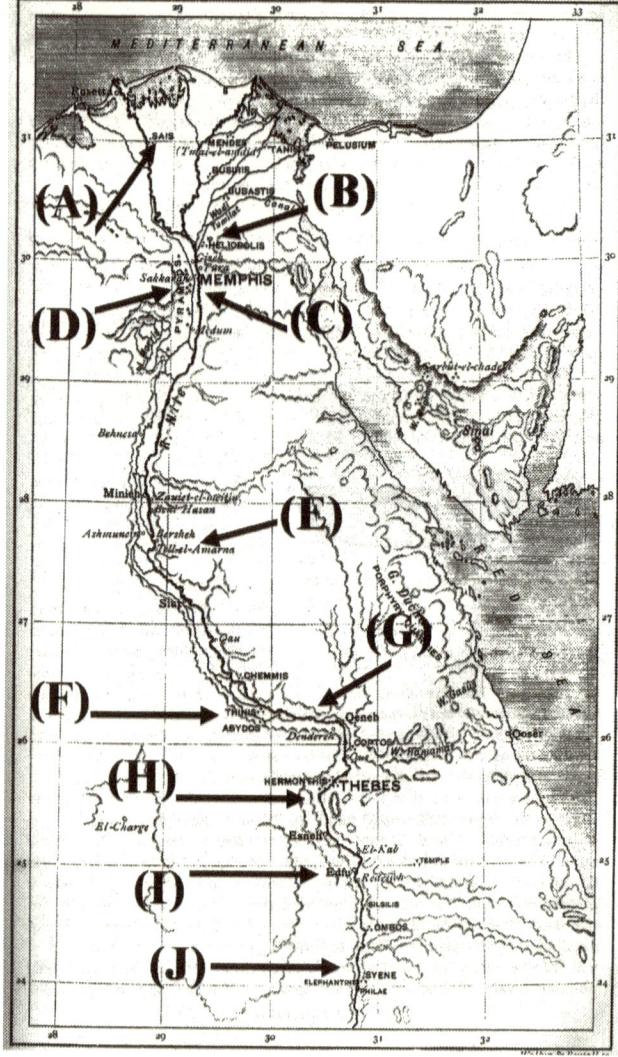

The Sphinx and its contemporary architecture throughout Kamit give us the earliest history, the earliest recorded evidence of the practice of advanced religion anywhere in the world. The Sphinx has now been proven to be the earliest example of the practice of religion in human history, 10,000 BCE.

The Ancient Egyptian Wisdom Texts

Before the Songai Empire
 Before Timbuktu
  Before the Mali Empire
  Before the Ghana Empire
  Before Islam
   Before Christianity
    Before the Sumerians
     Before the Greek Civilization
     Before the Roman Empire
    Before Hinduism
     Before Buddhism
    Before Europe
      Before The United States

THERE WAS KAMIT

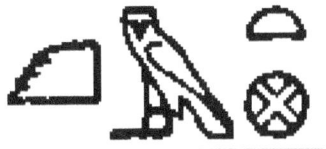

The Ancient Egyptian Wisdom Texts

When Was Ancient Egyptian Civilization?

A Brief History of Ancient Egypt

Christianity was partly an outgrowth of Judaism, which was itself an outgrowth of Ancient Egyptian culture and religion. So who were the Ancient Egyptians? From the time that the early Greek philosophers set foot on African soil to study the teachings of mystical spirituality in Egypt (900-300 B.C.E.), Western society and culture was forever changed. Ancient Egypt had such a profound effect on Western civilization as well as on the native population of Ancient India (Dravidians) that it is important to understand the history and culture of Ancient Egypt, and the nature of its spiritual tradition in more detail.

The history of Egypt begins in the far reaches of history. It includes The Dynastic Period, The Hellenistic Period, Roman and Byzantine Rule (30 B.C.E.-638 A.C.E.), the Caliphate and the Mamalukes (642-1517 A.C.E.), Ottoman Domination (1082-1882 A.C.E.), British colonialism (1882-1952 A.C.E.), as well as modern, Arab-Islamic Egypt (1952-present).

Ancient Egypt or Kamit, was a civilization that flourished in Northeast Africa along the Nile River from before 5,500 B.C.E. until 30 B.C.E. In 30 B.C.E., Octavian, who was later known as the Roman Emperor, Augustus, put the last Egyptian King, Ptolemy XIV, a Greek ruler, to death. After this Egypt was formally annexed to Rome. Egyptologists normally divide Ancient Egyptian history into the following periods: The Early Dynastic Period; The Old Kingdom or Old Empire; The First Intermediate Period; The Middle Kingdom or Middle Empire; The Second Intermediate Period; The New Kingdom or New Empire (1,532-1,070 B.C.E.); The third Intermediate Period (1,070-712 B.C.E.); The Late Period (712-332 B.C.E.).

In the Late Period the following groups controlled Egypt. The Nubian Dynasty (712-657 B.C.E.); The Persian Dynasty (525-404 B.C.E.); The Native Revolt and re-establishment of Egyptian rule by Egyptians (404-343 B.C.E.); The Second Persian Period (343-332 B.C.E.); The Ptolemaic or Greek Period (332 B.C.E.- c. 30 B.C.E.); Roman Period (c.30 B.C.E.-395 A.C.E.); The Byzantine Period (395-640 A.C.E) and The Arab

The Ancient Egyptian Wisdom Texts

Conquest Period (640 A.C.E.-present). The individual dynasties are numbered, generally in Roman numerals, from I through XXX. However, the realization of the geological evidence of the Great Sphinx and the discovery of the new Dynasty previously unknown to the Egyptologists, the history needs to be revised. See the full revision in the book African Origins of Civilization by Muata Ashby (2002).

The period after the New Kingdom saw greatness in culture and architecture under the rulership of Ramses II. However, after his rule, Egypt saw a decline from which it would never recover. This is the period of the downfall of Ancient Egyptian culture in which the Libyans ruled after the Tanite (XXI) Dynasty. This was followed by the Nubian conquerors who founded the XXII Dynasty and tried to restore Egypt to her past glory. However, having been weakened by the social and political turmoil of wars, Ancient Egypt fell to the Persians once more. The Persians conquered the country until the Greeks, under Alexander, conquered them. The Romans followed the Greeks, and finally the Arabs conquered the land of Egypt in 640 A.C.E to the present.

However, the history which has been classified above is only the history of the "Dynastic Period." It reflects the view of traditional Egyptologists who have refused to accept the evidence of a Predynastic period in Ancient Egyptian history contained in Ancient Egyptian documents such as the *Palermo Stone, Royal Tablets at Abydos, Royal Papyrus of Turin,* the *Dynastic List* of *Manetho,* and the eye-witness accounts of Greek historians Herodotus (c. 484-425 B.C.E.) and Diodorus. These sources speak clearly of a Pre-dynastic society which stretches far into antiquity. The Dynastic Period is what most people think of whenever Ancient Egypt is mentioned. This period is when the pharaohs (kings) ruled. The latter part of the Dynastic Period is when the Biblical story of Moses, Joseph, Abraham, etc., occurs (c. 2100? -1,000? B.C.E). Therefore, those with a Christian background generally only have an idea about Ancient Egypt as it is related in the Bible. The tradition based on the old Jewish bible recounting about how the Jews were used for forced labor and the construction of the great monuments of Egypt such as the Great Pyramids is impossible since these were created in the predynastic age, thousands of years before Abraham, the supposed first Jew, ever existed. Although this biblical notion is very limited in scope, the significant impact of Ancient Egypt on Hebrew and Christian culture is evident even from the biblical scriptures. Actually, Egypt existed much earlier than most traditional Egyptologists are prepared to admit. The new archeological evidence related to the great Sphinx monument on the Giza

The Ancient Egyptian Wisdom Texts

Plateau and the ancient writings by Manetho, one of the last High Priests of Ancient Egypt, show that Ancient Egyptian history begins earlier than 10,000 B.C.E. and may date back to as early as 30,000-50,000 B.C.E.

The Fundamental Principles of Ancient Egyptian Religion

NETERIANISM
(The Oldest Known Religion in History)

The term "Neterianism" is derived from the name "Shetaut Neter." Shetaut Neter means the "Hidden Divinity." It is the ancient philosophy and mythic spiritual culture that gave rise to the Ancient Egyptian civilization. Those who follow the spiritual path of Shetaut Neter are therefore referred to as "Neterians." The fundamental principles common to all denominations of Ancient Egyptian Religion may be summed up in four "Great Truths" that are common to all the traditions of Ancient Egyptian Religion.

The Ancient Egyptian Wisdom Texts

Summary of Ancient Egyptian Religion

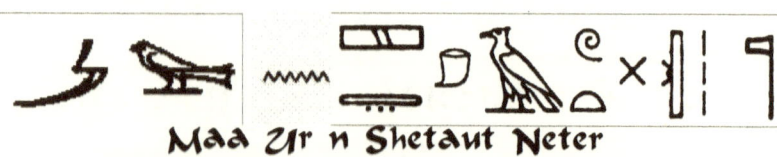

Maa Ur n Shetaut Neter
"Great Truths of The Shetaut Neter Religion"

I

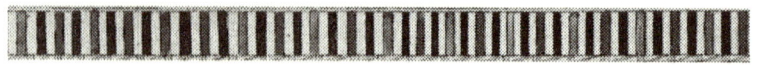

Pa Neter ua ua Neberdjer m Neteru
"The Neter, the Supreme Being, is One and alone and as Neberdjer, manifesting everywhere and in all things in the form of Gods and Goddesses."

II

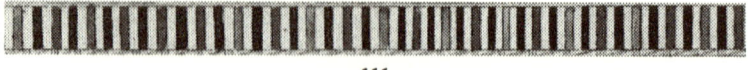

an-Maat swy Saui Set s-Khemn
"Lack of righteousness brings fetters to the personality and these fetters cause ignorance of the Divine."

III

16

The Ancient Egyptian Wisdom Texts

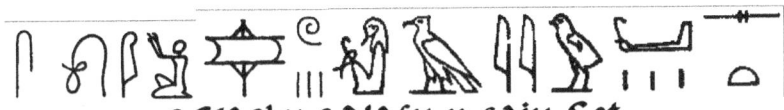

s-Uashu s-Nafu n saiu Set

"Devotion to the Divine leads to freedom from the fetters of Set."

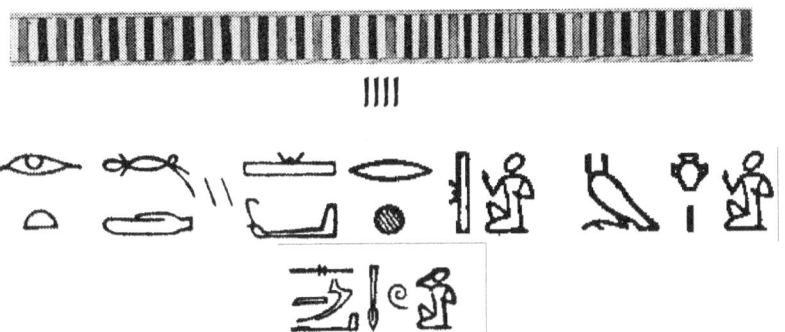

ari Shedy Rekh ab m Maakheru

"The practice of the Shedy disciplines leads to knowing oneself and the Divine. This is called being True of Speech"

The Ancient Egyptian Wisdom Texts

Neterian Great Truths

1. ***"Pa Neter ua ua Neberdjer m Neteru"*** -"The Neter, the Supreme Being, is One and alone and as Neberdjer, manifesting everywhere and in all things in the form of Gods and Goddesses."

Neberdjer means "all-encompassing divinity," the all-inclusive, all-embracing Spirit which pervades all and who is the ultimate essence of all. This first truth unifies all the expressions of Kamitan religion.

2. **"an-Maat swy Saui Set s-Khemn"** – "Lack of righteousness brings fetters to the personality and these fetters lead to ignorance of the Divine."

When a human being acts in ways that contradict the natural order of nature, negative qualities of the mind will develop within that person's personality. These are the afflictions of Set. Set is the neteru of egoism and selfishness. The afflictions of Set include: anger, hatred, greed, lust, jealousy, envy, gluttony, dishonesty, hypocrisy, etc. So to be free from the fetters of set one must be free from the afflictions of Set.

3. **"s-Uashu s-Nafu n saiu Set"** -"Devotion to the Divine leads to freedom from the fetters of Set."

To be liberated (Nafu - freedom - to breath) from the afflictions of Set, one must be devoted to the Divine. Being devoted to the Divine means living by Maat. Maat is a way of life that is purifying to the heart and beneficial for society as it promotes virtue and order. Living by Maat means practicing Shedy (spiritual practices and disciplines).

Uashu means devotion and the classic pose of adoring the Divine is called "Dua," standing or sitting with upraised hands facing outwards towards the image of the divinity.

The Ancient Egyptian Wisdom Texts

4. **"ari Shedy Rekh ab m Maakheru"** - "The practice of the Shedy disciplines leads to knowing oneself and the Divine. This is called being True of Speech."

Doing Shedy means to study profoundly, to penetrate the mysteries (Shetaut) and discover the nature of the Divine. There have been several practices designed by the sages of Ancient Kamit to facilitate the process of self-knowledge. These are the religious (Shetaut) traditions and the Sema (Smai) Tawi (yogic) disciplines related to them that augment the spiritual practices.

All the traditions relate the teachings of the sages by means of myths related to particular gods or goddesses. It is understood that all of these neteru are related, like brothers and sisters, having all emanated from the same source, the same Supremely Divine parent, who is neither male nor female, but encompasses the totality of the two.

The Ancient Egyptian Wisdom Texts

The Great Truths of Neterianism are realized by means of Four Spiritual Disciplines in Three Steps

The four disciples are: Rekh Shedy (Wisdom), Ari Shedy (Righteous Action and Selfless Service), Uashu (Ushet) Shedy (Devotion) and Uaa Shedy (Meditation)

The Spiritual Culture and the Purpose of Life: Shetaut Neter

"Men and women are to become God-like
through a life of virtue and the cultivation of
the spirit through scientific knowledge,
practice and bodily discipline."

-Ancient Egyptian Proverb

The highest forms of Joy, Peace and Contentment are obtained when the meaning of life is discovered. When the human being is in harmony with life, then it is possible to reflect and meditate upon the human condition and realize the limitations of worldly pursuits. When there is peace and harmony in life, a human being can practice any of the varied disciplines designated as Shetaut Neter to promote {his/her} evolution towards the ultimate goal of life, which Spiritual Enlightenment. Spiritual Enlightenment is the awakening of a human being to the awareness of the Transcendental essence which binds the universe and which is eternal and immutable. In this discovery is also the sobering and ecstatic realization that the human being is one with that Transcendental essence. With this realization comes great joy, peace and power to experience the fullness of life and to realize the purpose of life during the time on earth. The lotus is a symbol of Shetaut Neter, meaning the turning towards the light of truth, peace and transcendental harmony.

Shetaut Neter

We have established that the Ancient Egyptians were African peoples who lived in the north-eastern quadrant of the continent of Africa. They were descendants of the Nubians, who had themselves originated from farther south into the heart of Africa at the Great Lakes region, the sources of the Nile River. They created a vast civilization and culture earlier than any other society in known history and organized a nation that was based

The Ancient Egyptian Wisdom Texts

on the concepts of balance and order as well as spiritual enlightenment. These ancient African people called their land Kamit, and soon after developing a well-ordered society, they began to realize that the world is full of wonders, but also that life is fleeting, and that there must be something more to human existence. They developed spiritual systems that were designed to allow human beings to understand the nature of this secret being who is the essence of all Creation. They called this spiritual system "Shtaut Ntr (Shetaut Neter)."

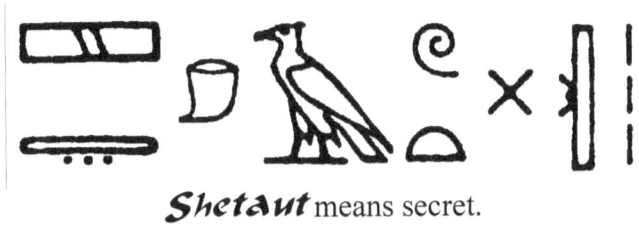

Shetaut means secret.

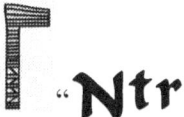

Neter means Divinity.
Who is Neter in Kamitan Religion?

"**Ntr**

The symbol of Neter was described by an Ancient Kamitan priest as:
"That which is placed in the coffin"

The term Ntr, or Ntjr, comes from the Ancient Egyptian hieroglyphic language which did not record its vowels. However, the term survives in the Coptic language as *"Nutar."* The same Coptic meaning (divine force or sustaining power) applies in the present as it did in ancient times. It is a symbol composed of a wooden staff that was wrapped with strips of fabric, like a mummy. The strips alternate in color with yellow, green and blue. The mummy in Kamitan spirituality is understood to be the dead but resurrected Divinity. So the Nutar (Ntr) is actually every human being who does not really die, but goes to live on in a different form. Further, the resurrected spirit of every human being is that same Divinity. Phonetically, the term Nutar is related to other terms having the same meaning, such as the latin "Natura," the Spanish Naturalesa, the English "Nature" and "Nutriment", etc. In a real sense, as we will see, Natur means power manifesting as Neteru and the Neteru are the objects of creation, i.e. "nature."

The Great Awakening of Neterian Religion

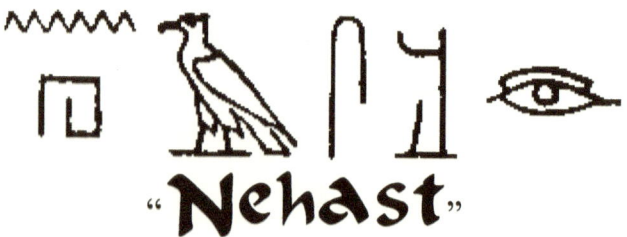

"Nehast"

Nehast means to "wake up," to Awaken to the higher existence. In the Prt m Hru Text it is said:

Nuk pa Neter aah Neter Ua asha ren

"I am that same God, the Supreme One, who has myriad of mysterious names."

The goal of all the Neterian disciplines is to discover the meaning of "Who am I?," to unravel the mysteries of life and to fathom the depths of eternity and infinity. This is the task of all human beings and it is to be accomplished in this very lifetime.

---

[1] (Prt M Hru 9:4)

The Ancient Egyptian Wisdom Texts

This can be done by learning the ways of the Neteru, emulating them and finally becoming like them, Akhus, (enlightened beings), walking the earth as giants and accomplishing great deeds such as the creation of the universe!

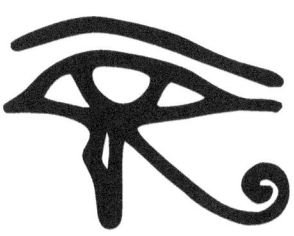

Udjat

The Eye of Heru is a quintessential symbol of awakening to Divine Consciousness, representing the concept of Nehast.

The Ancient Egyptian Wisdom Texts

Sacred Scriptures of Shetaut Neter

The following scriptures represent the foundational scriptures of Kamitan culture. They may be divided into three categories: *Mythic Scriptures*, *Mystical Philosophy* and *Ritual Scriptures*, and *Wisdom Scriptures* (Didactic Literature).

MYTHIC SCRIPTURES Literature	Mystical (Ritual) Philosophy Literature	Wisdom Texts Literature
Shetaut Asar-Aset-Heru The Myth of Asar, Aset and Heru (Asarian Resurrection Theology) - Predynastic Shetaut Atum-Ra Anunian Theology Predynastic Shetaut Net/Aset/Hetheru Saitian Theology – Goddess Spirituality Predynastic Shetaut Ptah Memphite Theology Predynastic Shetaut Amun Theban Theology Predynastic	**Coffin Texts** (C. 2040 B.C.E.-1786 B.C.E.) **Papyrus Texts** (C. 1580 B.C.E.-Roman Period)[2] Books of Coming Forth By Day Example of famous papyri: Papyrus of Any Papyrus of Hunefer Papyrus of Kenna Greenfield Papyrus, Etc.	**Wisdom Texts** (C. 3,000 B.C.E. – PTOLEMAIC PERIOD) Precepts of Ptahotep Instructions of Any Instructions of Amenemope Etc. Hermetic Texts **Maat Declarations** Literature (All Periods) Blind Harpers Songs

---

[2] After 1570 B.C.E they would evolve into a more unified text, the Egyptian Book of the Dead.

The Ancient Egyptian Wisdom Texts

Neter and the Neteru

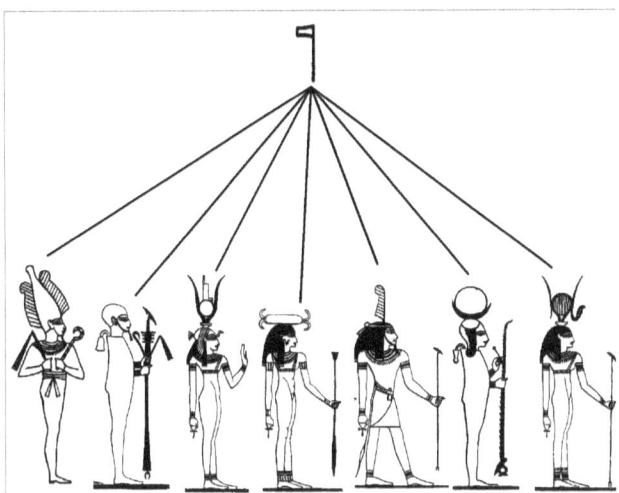

The Neteru (Gods and Goddesses) proceed from the Neter (Supreme Being)

As stated earlier, the concept of Neter and Neteru binds and ties all of the varied forms of Kamitan spirituality into one vision of the gods and goddesses all emerging from the same Supreme Being. Therefore, ultimately, Kamitan spirituality is not polytheistic, nor is it monotheistic, for it holds that the Supreme Being is more than a God or Goddess. The Supreme Being is an all-encompassing Absolute Divinity.

The Neteru

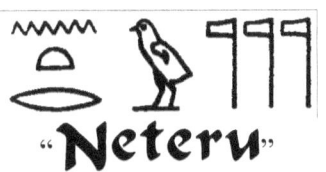

The term "Neteru" means "gods and goddesses." This means that from the ultimate and transcendental Supreme Being, "Neter," come the Neteru. There are countless Neteru. So from the one come the many. These Neteru are cosmic forces that pervade the universe. They are the means by which

The Ancient Egyptian Wisdom Texts

Neter sustains Creation and manifests through it. So Neterianism is a monotheistic polytheism. The one Supreme Being expresses as many gods and goddesses. At the end of time, after their work of sustaining Creation is finished, these gods and goddesses are again absorbed back into the Supreme Being.

All of the spiritual systems of Ancient Egypt (Kamit) have one essential aspect that is common to all; they all hold that there is a Supreme Being (Neter) who manifests in a multiplicity of ways through nature, the Neteru. Like sunrays, the Neteru emanate from the Divine; they are its manifestations. So by studying the Neteru we learn about and are led to discover their source, the Neter, and with this discovery we are enlightened. The Neteru may be depicted anthropomorphically or zoomorphically in accordance with the teaching about Neter that is being conveyed through them.

The Ancient Egyptian Wisdom Texts

The General Principles of Shetaut Neter (Teachings Presented in the Kamitan scriptures)

1. The Purpose of Life is to Attain the Great Awakening-Enlightenment-Know thyself.

2. SHETAUT NETER enjoins the Shedy (spiritual investigation) as the highest endeavor of life.

3. SHETAUT NETER enjoins that it is the responsibility of every human being to promote order and truth.

4. SHETAUT NETER enjoins the performance of Selfless Service to family, community and humanity.

5. SHETAUT NETER enjoins the Protection of nature.

6. SHETAUT NETER enjoins the Protection of the weak and oppressed.

7. SHETAUT NETER enjoins the Caring for hungry.

8. SHETAUT NETER enjoins the Caring for homeless.

9. SHETAUT NETER enjoins the equality for all people.

10. SHETAUT NETER enjoins the equality between men and women.

11. SHETAUT NETER enjoins the justice for all.

12. SHETAUT NETER enjoins the sharing of resources.

13. SHETAUT NETER enjoins the protection and proper raising of children.

14. SHETAUT NETER enjoins the movement towards balance and peace.

The Ancient Egyptian Wisdom Texts

Medu Neter

"Medu Neter"

The teachings of the Neterian Traditions are conveyed in the scriptures of the Neterian Traditions. These are recorded in the Medu Neter script.

Hieroglyphic Script

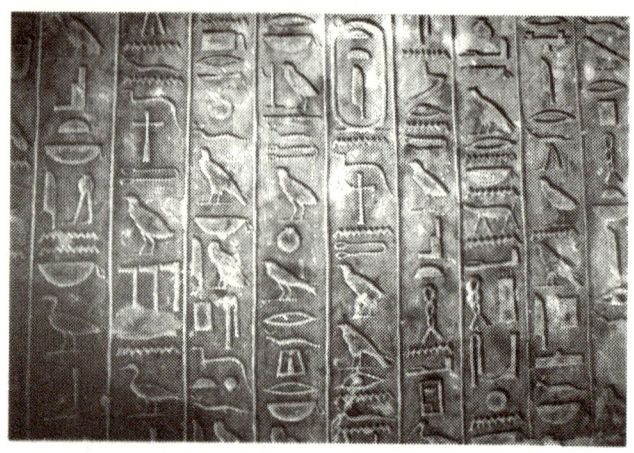

Above: A section from the pyramid of Teti in Sakkara Egypt, known as the "Pyramid Texts" (Early Dynastic Period) showing the cross

The Medu Neter was used through all periods by Priests and priestesses – mostly used in monumental inscriptions such as the Pyramid texts, Obelisks, temple inscriptions, etc. – since Pre-Dynastic times. It is the earliest form of writing in known history.

The Ancient Egyptian Wisdom Texts

Hekau, Medu Neter and Shetitu as Vehicles of the Wisdom Teachings

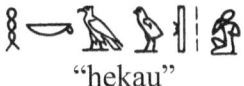
"hekau"

The concept of the divine word or *Hekau,* is an extremely important part of Ancient Egyptian religion and is instructive in the study of all African religion. The only difference between Ancient Egyptian religion and other African religions in this area was the extensive development of the "written word." As explained earlier, the word religion is translated as Shetaut Neter in the Ancient African language of Kamit.

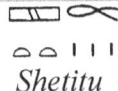
Shetitu

This Shetaut (mysteries- rituals, wisdom, philosophy) about the Neter (Supreme Being) are related in the ▱◦◦|||*Shetitu* or writings related to the hidden teaching. And those writings are referred to as 𓎸𓏛 *Medu Neter* or "Divine Speech," the writings of the god Djehuti (Ancient Egyptian god of the divine word) – also refers to any hieroglyphic texts or inscriptions generally. The term Medu Neter makes use of a special hieroglyph, 𓌁, which means "*medu*" or "staff - walking stick-speech." This means that speech is the support for the Divine, 𓌁. Thus, just as the staff supports an elderly person, the hieroglyphic writing (the word) is a prop (staff) which sustains the Divine in the realm of time and space. That is, the Divine writings contain the wisdom which enlightens us about the Divine, ▱◦𓆼𓄿×𓀀 𓌁*Shetaut Neter.*

If Medu Neter is mastered then the spiritual aspirant becomes 𓌳𓐙𓏤𓊤 Maakheru or true of thought, word and deed, that

The Ancient Egyptian Wisdom Texts

is, purified in body, mind and soul. The symbol medu is static while the symbol of Kheru is dynamic.

This term (Maakheru) uses the glyph ◊ kheru is a rudder – oar (rowing), symbol of voice, meaning that purification occurs when the righteous movement of the word, when it is used (rowing-movement) to promote virtue, order, peace, harmony and truth. So Medu Neter is the potential word and Maa kheru is the perfected word.

The hieroglyphic texts (Medu Neter) become (Maakheru) useful in the process of religion when they are used as 𓎡𓄿𓅱𓏏𓏤𓀁 hekau - the Ancient Egyptian "Words of Power" when the word is 𓎛𓋴𓇋𓀁 Hesi, chanted and 𓆈𓇋𓏤𓀁 Shmai- sung and thereby one performs ★𓀀 or ★𓅓𓀢 Dua or worship of the Divine. The divine word allows the speaker to control the gods and goddesses, i.e. the cosmic forces. This concept is really based on the idea that human beings are higher order beings if they learn about the nature of the universe and elevate themselves through virtue and wisdom.

Ancient Egyptian Proverbs On The Purpose of Life and the Value of Wisdom Teachings

"The many do confound philosophy with multifarious reasoning... by mixing it, by means of subtle expositions, with diverse sciences not easy to be grasped-such as arithmetic, and music, and geometry. But pure philosophy, which doth depend on Godly piety alone, should only so far occupy itself with other arts, that it may appreciate the working out in numbers of the fore-appointed stations of the stars when they return, and of the course of their procession...know how to appreciate the Earth's dimensions, qualities and quantities, the Water's depths, the strength of Fire, and the effect and nature of all these...give worship and give praise unto the Art and Mind of God."

"Wisdom is a child of training; Truth is the child of Wisdom and Love."

"Death comes when the purpose of living is fulfilled; death shows what the reason for living was."

The Ancient Egyptian Wisdom Texts

"Scorn also to depress thy competitor by any dishonest or unworthy method; strive to raise thyself above them by excelling them; so shall thy contest for superiority to be crowned with honor, if not with success."

"If the social order judges success by material gain, the most successful will be the most corruptible and selfish."

"Accurate reckoning (mathematics), the entrance into the knowledge of all existing things and all obscure secrets."

"If you meet a disputant who is not your equal or match, do not attack, they are weak. They will confound themselves. Do not answer the evil speech and give in to your animal passion for combat by venting your self against them. You will beat them through the reproof of the witnesses who will agree with you."

"What is the pay for titles, but flattery? How doth man purchase power but by being a slave to him who giveth it?"

"Magic is knowledge and strength; without strength, nothing worthwhile can be achieved, without knowledge, strength is uncontrolled."

"As above, so below; as below, so above."
"The mover must have greater power than the moved."

The Ancient Egyptian Wisdom Texts

"All that exists on earth is an incarnation of the real essence from the non-material realm."

"Courage, will, knowledge and silence are essential qualities for those on the path of perfection."

"They who began to benefit from words of wisdom while they were children shall prosper in their affairs."

"Men and women are to become God-like through a life of virtue and the cultivation of the spirit through scientific knowledge, practice and bodily discipline."

"Salvation is the freeing of the soul from its bodily fetters; becoming a God through knowledge and wisdom; controlling the forces of the cosmos instead of being a slave to them; subduing the lower nature and through awakening the higher self, ending the cycle of rebirth and dwelling with the Neters who direct and control the Great Plan."

-Ancient Egyptian Proverbs

The Ancient Egyptian Wisdom Texts

How to Be a Worthy Aspirant to be Admitted to the Wisdom Teachings

The Wisdom Texts are philosophical wisdom teachings that are to be listended to. They are to be espoused by a qualified spiritual preceptor and the aspirant needs to cultivate certain qualities in order to be inducted into the ranks of the few qualified initiates able to sit at the feet of spiritual masters. This writing recalls the teaching of the Greek Aspirant, a story about a Greek man who sought to be taught by an Ancient Egyptian sage. The Greek aspirant ultimately proved unworthy of the teacher but his wrong actions inform us of the deficiencies of spiritual aspirants so we may avoid those on the spiritual path. The following story was written by Lucian, called *Philopseudes,* about a sacred scribe of Memphis (Ancient Egyptian city Menefer) and the misadventures of his hero Eucrates:

The Greek Aspirant

"In my youth, when I was living in Egypt-my father sent me there to finish my education-I thought it would be nice to sail up the Nile as far as Coptus, travel on from there to the statue of Memnon and hear the strange sound that it makes at sunrise. Well I heard it all right, but it was not just the meaningless noise that most people hear. On the contrary, Memnon actually opened his mouth and gave me a seven-line oracle in verse, which I could repeat to you word for word, if there were any point in doing so. On the voyage back, one of my fellow-passengers was a holy scribe from Memphis, an incredibly wise man who'd mastered all the mystic lore of Egypt. He was said to have lived for twenty-three years in an underground shrine, receiving instruction in magic from Isis."
"Why that sounds like the man that taught me!" exclaimed Arignotus.
"Pancrates, his name was-a very holy man, clean-shaven, always wore linen, highly intelligent, spoke rather bad Greek, tallish, snub nose, thick lips, and rather thin legs."

The Ancient Egyptian Wisdom Texts

"Yes, Pancrates! That's exactly who it was," said Eucrates. "I'd never heard of him before, but when I saw the amazing things he did every time we landed, like riding about on crocodiles and going for swims with them-when I saw the great brutes crouching at his feet and wagging their tails, I realized that he must be a Holy Man. Very gradually, by various small acts of courtesy, I managed to make friends with him and he told me all his secrets. Finally he persuaded me to leave my own employees at Memphis, and go off with him. He said there wouldn't be any problem about servants. So off we went.
"Whenever we stopped at an inn, he used to take a broom, or a rolling-pin, or the bolt off the door, dress it up, and then, by saying, a spell, make it walk about just like a human being.

It went and fetched us hot water, did all the shopping and the cooking, and generally acted as a most efficient domestic servant. When there was nothing more for it to do, he'd say another spell, which turned it back into a broom, or a rolling pin, as the case might be. Much as I wanted to, I could never get him to show me how he did it, for he was very jealous of this particular accomplishment, though he was quite prepared to tell me everything else.
"However, one day I hid in a dark corner while he was doing it, and overheard the spell-it was only three syllables long. Having told the rolling-pin what he wanted done, he went off into the town. So next day, when he again had business in town, I seized the rolling-pin, dressed it up, pronounced the three syllables, and told it to fetch some water. When it came back with a bucketful, I said: 'That'll do. Don't fetch any more water, but turn back into a rolling-pin.' This time it refused to obey me, but went on fetching bucket after bucket of water, until the whole house was flooded. I couldn't think what to do, for I was afraid Pancrates would be rather annoyed when he got back-as indeed he was. In despair, I seized an axe and chopped the rolling-pin in two whereupon each half grabbed a bucket and went on fetching water, so now I had twice as much water coming in! At this point Pancrates turned up, and realizing what had happened, turned both halves back into wood again. He then abandoned me in disgust, and mysteriously disappeared."

The story above contains important instructions on how to approach the Ancient Egyptian master, with patience, respect, purity and humility. Without these mature qualities of personality, an aspirant cannot learn the teaching and realize the wondrous nature of the mysteries. Many times people come to the teachings desiring immediate enlightenment and therefore not being willing to spend the time and applying themselves diligently to studying the philosophy and practicing the disciplines enjoined.

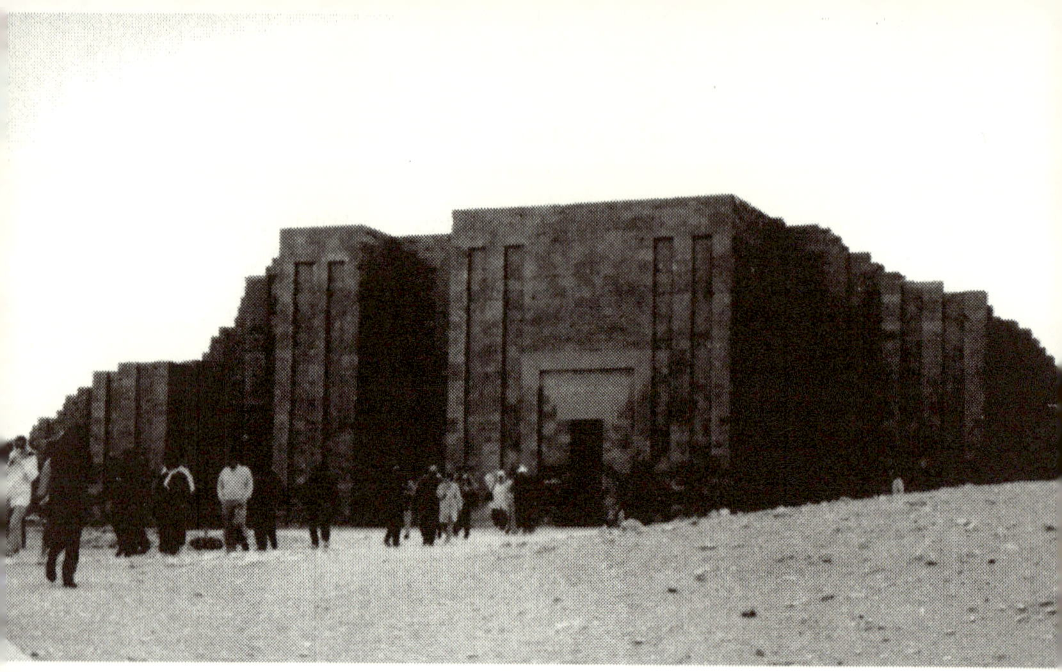

Above: Main entrance to the ancient Spiritual Center and Temple of Memphis at Sakkara, Egypt, the city where the Greek Aspirant Found the Ancient Egyptian Master.

Below: reconstructed section of the main temple at the Djozer complex in Sakkara Egypt {Menefer-Memphis}

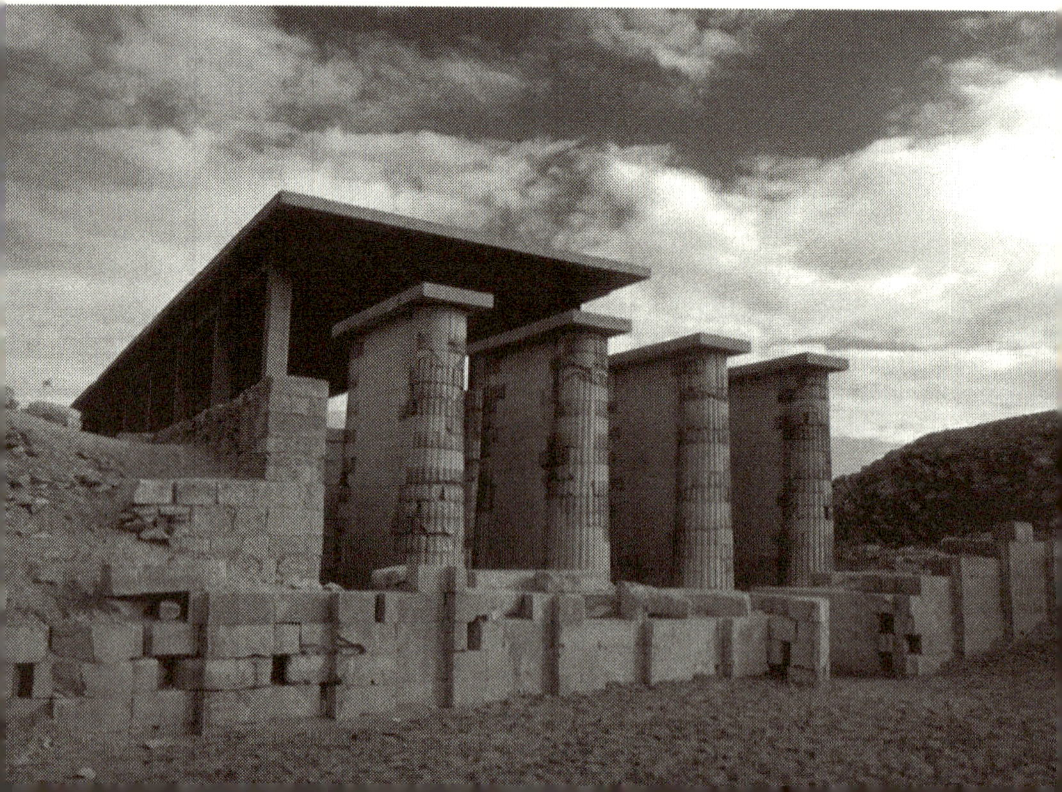

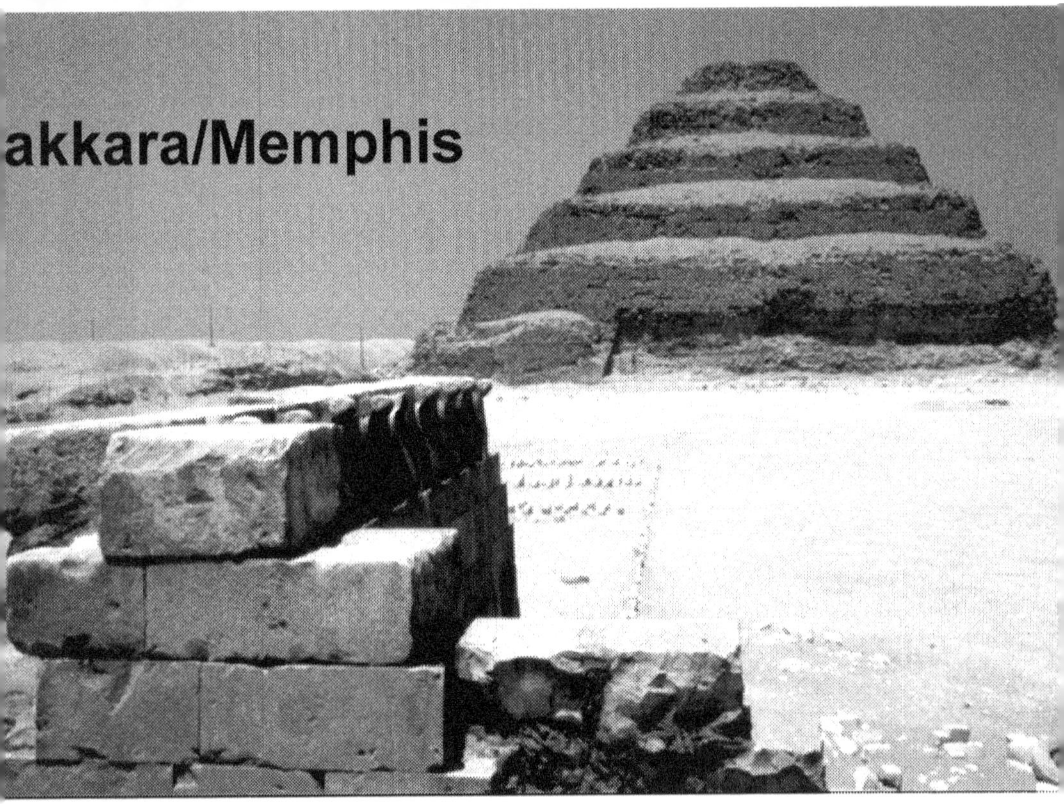

Sakkara/Memphis

Above: *Djozer Pyramid Complex* with the *Step Pyramid of Imhotep* located in Sakkara, Egypt– From the Old Kingdom Period – Third Dynasty- School of Memphite Theology- based on the Divinity *Ptah*.

Below: Ptah, the God of Menefer

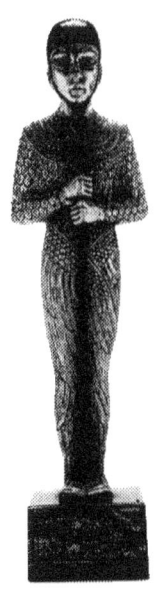

The Ancient Egyptian Wisdom Texts

How to Listen, Reflect and Meditate on the Wisdom Teachings

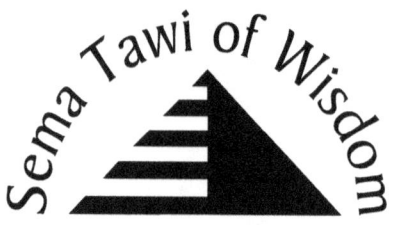

Listening to the Teachings

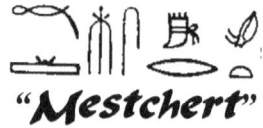

"Listening, to fill the ears, listen attentively-"

What should the ears be filled with?

The sages of Shetaut Neter enjoined that a Shemsu Neter (follower of Neter, an initiate or aspirant) should listen to the WISDOM of the Neterian Traditions. These are the myth related to the gods and goddesses containing the basic understanding of who they are, what they represent, how they relate human beings and to the Supreme Being. The myths allow us to be connected to the Divine.

The Ancient Egyptian Wisdom Texts

THE THREE-FOLD PROCESS OF WISDOM YOGA IN EGYPT:

According to the teachings of *the Ancient Temple of Aset* the Mysteries discipline of Wisdom, entails the process of three steps:

Discipline of Wisdom Philosophy in Ancient Egypt

1-<u>Listening</u> to the wisdom teachings on the nature of reality (creation) and the nature of the Self.

2-<u>Reflecting</u> on those teachings and incorporating them into daily life.

3-<u>Meditating</u> on the meaning of the teachings.

In the Temple of Aset (Aset) in Ancient Egypt the Discipline of the Yoga of Wisdom is imparted in three stages:

1-<u>Listening</u> to the wisdom teachings on the nature of reality (creation) and the nature of the Self.
2-<u>Reflecting</u> on those teachings and incorporating them into daily life.
3-<u>Meditating</u> on the meaning of the teachings.

Aset (Aset) was and is recognized as the goddess of wisdom and her temple strongly emphasized and espoused the philosophy of wisdom teaching in order to achieve higher spiritual consciousness. It is important to note here that the teaching which was practiced in the Ancient Egyptian Temple of Aset[3] of **Listening** to, **Reflecting** upon, and **Meditating** upon the teachings. **The Yoga of Wisdom** is a form of Yoga based on insight into the nature of worldly existence and the transcendental Self, thereby transforming one's consciousness through development of the wisdom

---

[3] See the book *The Wisdom of* Aset by Dr. Muata Ashby

faculty. Thus, we have here a correlation between Ancient Egypt that matches exactly in its basic factor respects.

Figure: The image of goddess Aset (Aset) suckling the young king is the quintessential symbol of initiation in Ancient Egypt.

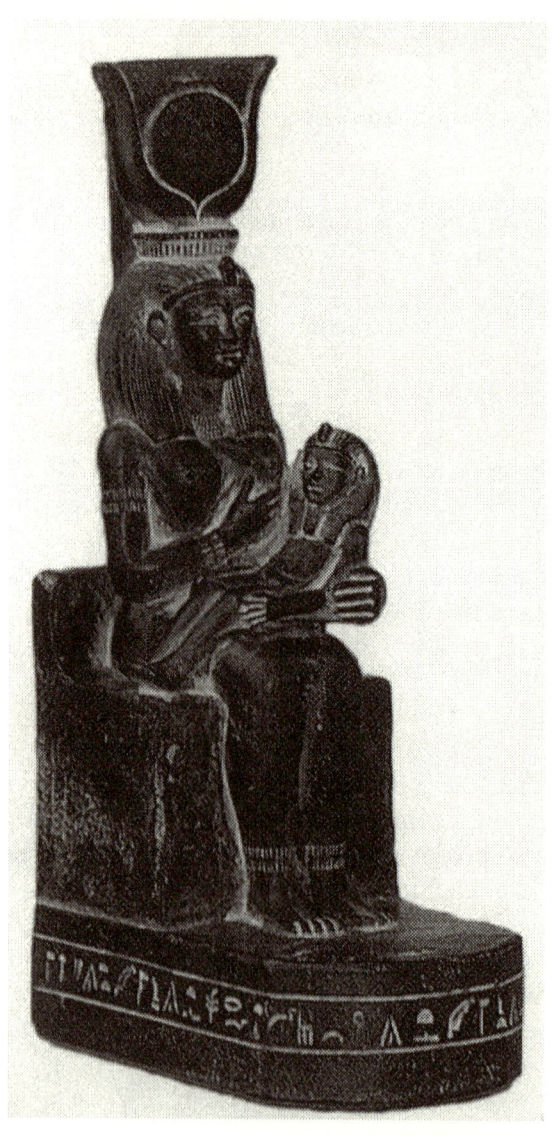

The Ancient Egyptian Wisdom Texts

Temple of Aset
GENERAL DISCIPLINE

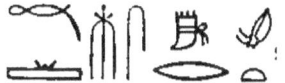

Fill the ears, listen attentively- Meh mestchert.

Listening

1- Listening to Wisdom teachings. Having achieved the qualifications of an aspirant, there is a desire to listen to the teachings from a Spiritual Preceptor. There is increasing intellectual understanding of the scriptures and the meaning of truth versus untruth, real versus unreal, temporal versus eternal. The glories of God are expounded and the mystical philosophy behind the myth is given at this stage.

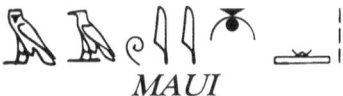
MAUI

"to think, to ponder, to fix attention, concentration"

Reflection

2- Reflection on those teachings that have been listened to and living according to the disciplines enjoined by the teachings is to be practiced until the wisdom teaching is fully understood. Reflection implies discovering, intellectually at first, the oneness behind the multiplicity of the world by engaging in intense inquiry into the nature of one's true Self. Chanting the hekau and divine singing *Hesi,* are also used here.

"Devote yourself to adore God's name."
—Ancient Egyptian Proverb

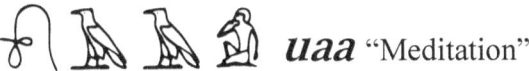 *uaa* "Meditation"

Meditation

3- Meditation in Wisdom Yoga is the process of reflection that leads to a state in which the mind is continuously introspective. It means expansion of consciousness culminating in revelation of and identification with the Absolute Self.

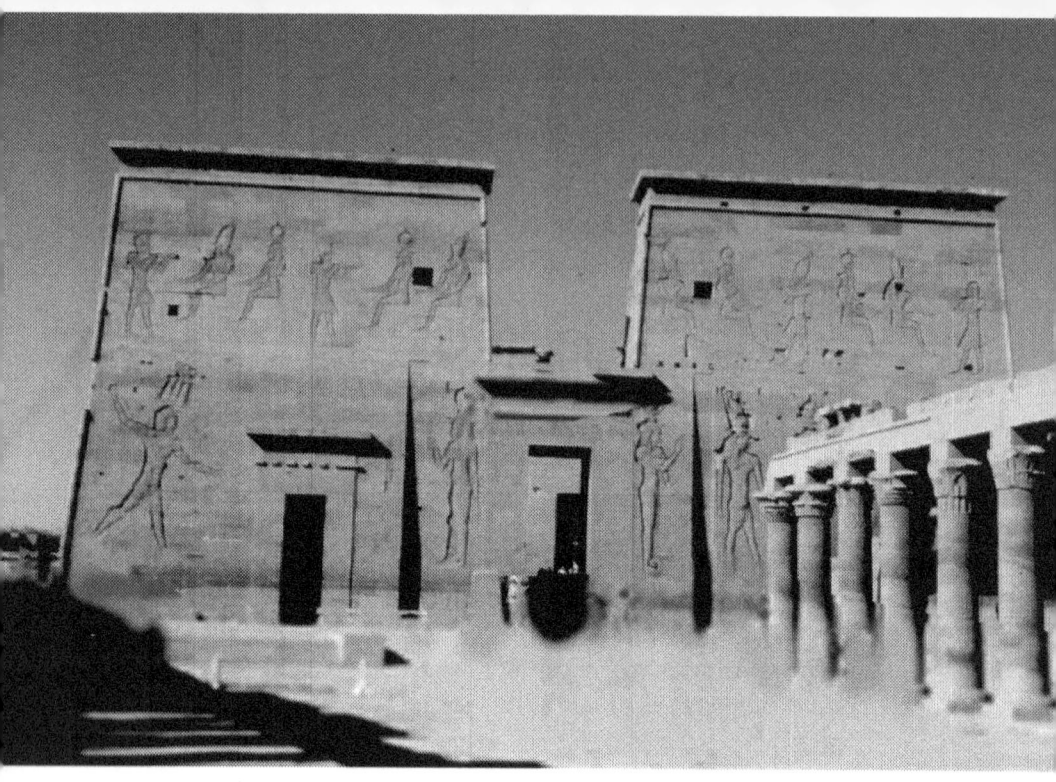
Above: Temple of Aset (Isis), where the wisdom of Listening, Reflecting and Meditation was taught in ancient times.

The Significance of the Ancient Egyptian Wisdom Texts

INTRODUCTION

The Ancient Egyptian Wisdom Texts are a genre of writings from the ancient culture that have survived to the present and provide a vibrant record of the practice of spiritual evolution otherwise known as religion or yoga philosophy in Ancient Egypt. The principle focus of the Wisdom Texts is the cultivation of understanding, peace, harmony, selfless service, self-control, Inner fulfillment and spiritual realization. When these factors are cultivated in human life, the virtuous qualities in a human being begin to manifest and sinfulness, ignorance and negativity diminish until a person is able to enter into higher consciousness, the coveted goal of all civilizations. It is this virtuous mode of life which opens the door to self-discovery and spiritual enlightenment. Therefore, the Wisdom Texts are important scriptures on the subject of human nature, spiritual psychology and mystical philosophy.

The teachings presented in the Wisdom Texts form the foundation of religion as well as the guidelines for conducting the affairs of every area of social interaction including commerce, education, the army, marriage, and especially the legal system. These texts were sources for the famous 42 Precepts of Maat of the Pert M Heru (Book of the Dead), essential regulations of good conduct to develop virtue and purity in order to attain higher consciousness and immortality after death.

Sections of the Wisdom Texts were used in ancient times as writing exercises for children learning to read and write, so instead of learning to write with meaningless sentences the teachers used the wisdom teachings to impart spiritual wisdom philosophy at the same time as the capacity to read and write.

The Ancient Egyptian Wisdom Texts

Every judge in Ancient Egypt was a priest or priestess of Maat or the Neter (deity) who presides over truth, justice, righteousness and order. Therefore, in Ancient Egypt there was no concept of separation of church and state as in modern times. The Ancient Egyptians recognized that all phenomena in nature as well as all phenomena in human experience are related to a reality which transcends ordinary human experience and perception. Therefore, how could it be possible to carry on as if the phenomenal world simply came into existence by chance and owes its existence to nothing and is supported by nothing, it just is. Such notions would have been understood by the Ancient Egyptians as expressions of spiritual ignorance. Thus, every area of Ancient Egyptian culture affirmed and acknowledged the Divine presence and the Wisdom Texts sought to assist human beings in living according to that Divine essence so as to discover it in its true form. So righteousness and virtue are essential aspects of the spiritual path in themselves which allow a human being to create peace and harmony in secular life and to discover a higher spiritual reality in the non-secular life.

What is Virtue?

The American Heritage Dictionary defines *Virtue* as:

> "Moral excellence and righteousness; goodness."

Virtue is the primary concern of the Wisdom Texts. What is virtue and where does it come from? Is it something which may be purchased? Is it something that can be cultivated? A person may be ordered to be obedient, to follow rules, etc. Is this virtue? If the Ten Commandments and so many other laws are established in society, why then is it that there is increasing crime and increasing strife among people? Why is there enmity in the world? Why is there a desire to hurt others? Why is there a desire to misappropriate the property of others?

Anger and hatred cannot be stopped by simply telling someone to be good, loving, forgiving and so on. One cannot become righteous by being ordered to or forced to, no more than a plant can be forced to grow, bear

The Ancient Egyptian Wisdom Texts

fruit or flowers through a command by the farmer. One can be compelled to follow rules but this does not mean that one is necessarily a virtuous person. Many people do not commit crimes and yet they are not virtuous because they are harboring negative thoughts (violence, hatred, greed, lust, etc.) in their hearts. Virtue is a profound quality which every human being has a potential to discover. However, this requires effort on the part of the individual as well as the correct guidance. Virtue is like a flower which can grow and become beautiful for the whole world to see. However, just as a plant must receive the proper nutrients (soil, water, sunlight, etc.) so too the human heart must receive the proper caring and nurturing in the form of love, wisdom, proper diet, meditation and good will.

Many people are law abiding and peaceful under normal conditions, but if provoked or presented with an opportunity, they will engage in unrighteous activity. Under pressure they may be pushed into stealing, violence or other vices. This is not virtue. The development of virtue in a human being implies that sinful behavior will not be possible even if there is an opportunity for it. True virtue implies a profound understanding of the nature of creation and the heart which will make it impossible to commit crimes or to consider sinful thoughts; as we discover the teachings of Maat, the reasons for this will become clear.

Virtue is the quality which implies harmony with the universe. Virtue is that which leads a human being to come into harmony with the Divine. From a mythological standpoint, sin is to be understood as the absence of wisdom which leads to righteousness and peace and the existence of ignorance which leads to mental unrest and the endless desires of the mind. Sin operates in human life as any movement which works against self-discovery, and virtue is any movement towards discovering the essential truth of the innermost heart. The state of ignorance will end only when the mind develops a higher vision. It must look beyond the illusions of human desire and begin to seek something more substantial and abiding. This is when the aspirant develops an interest in spirituality and the practice of order, correctness, self-improvement and intellectual development. In ancient Egyptian Mythology and mystical philosophy, these qualities are symbolized by the Deities MAAT and Anpu (Anubis). Maat is the truth and Anpu is the symbol of the discerning intellect which can see right from wrong, good from evil, truth from untruth, etc.

The Ancient Egyptian Wisdom Texts

It must be clearly understood that vicious behavior or behaviors that are based on pursuing vices, is/are a factor of spiritual immaturity. Every human being has the innate capacity to develop and experience a virtuous character. Therefore, if one wants to promote peace and non-violence in the world, one must seek to promote virtue in others. This means helping others to discover their inner potential for experiencing a higher state of connectedness to humanity and the universe and a deeper fulfillment in life. Anger and violence are the mark of immaturity. Those who seek to use violence to have their way, to control others, or to promote order in society are in reality expressing their own inability to control themselves. When there is true virtue there will be no desire to control others for egoistic purposes or through the use of violence. A person of strong virtuous character will be able to control himself / herself so as to exercise great care and patience with others. This virtuous development allows a human being to develop a strong will and exert a strong influence on others which can be used to direct them toward what is positive and good. This kind of spiritual power was demonstrated by great Sages and Saints throughout history (Imhotep, Ptahotep, Osiris, Isis, Buddha, Jesus, Krishna, etc.). All of the Sages and Saints just mentioned are no different than any other human being who ever existed, except in the lifestyle they chose to live. They chose to live in such a way that the negative in them was eradicated and the wisdom of self-discovery was allowed to blossom. This is the path of virtue wherein life is lived for purifying the mind and body so as to allow the Higher Self, the Spirit in the heart, to emerge and be discovered.

In order to gain this form of spiritual power and spiritual enlightenment, it is necessary to root out every bit of ignorance and negativity in one's entire being. This means that there must be a clear insight into the nature of one's own spiritual innermost nature. This also means that one's actions, thoughts and words must be pure. When the path of virtue is perfected, the heights of spiritual wisdom illuminate the heart. This is the meaning of MAAT Philosophy. Maat is a path of life which leads to spiritual Enlightenment through the Path of Virtue.

The main concern of the Ancient Egyptian Wisdom Texts is the teaching of a way of live which promotes truth, non-violence, self-control

The Ancient Egyptian Wisdom Texts

and righteous action, balance of mind, and sublimation of egoistic and sexual desires.

The Wisdom Texts are ancient Egyptian writings which extol the virtue of righteous living and the idea of righteous living as a path to spiritual enlightenment. We will explore two of the most important forms of the wisdom texts which are representative of the form of writing. The main purpose of the texts is to instruct in the art of living which leads to peace and harmony in life and spiritual emancipation through effacement of the ego and devotion to God.

Though the Pert M Hru (Ancient Egyptian Book of Coming Forth By Day, Book of the Dead) is the most popular text of Ancient Egypt it will be soon realized that the Wisdom Texts are the source of the teachings presented in the Book of Coming Forth By Day. The teachings expressed in the Book of Coming Forth By Day known as the 42 precepts of Maat are in reality a culmination or an affirmation of a life lived according to righteous conduct and spiritual wisdom. The Wisdom Texts date back to the period of 5,000 B.C.E. known as the "Old Kingdom" period of Dynastic Egypt and represent the earliest known examples of instructions in the art of living for harmony in society and for spiritual evolution. They were copied upon papyri (paper) and were designed for the general instruction of the Ancient Egyptian population.

In Chapter 125 of the Ancient Egyptian Book of Coming Forth By Day it is stated that one should be able to declare one's innocence from wrong doing in order to see the face of God. How is this possible? Can a human being aspire to perfection and divine vision? The Wisdom Texts show how this is possible in language and instructions which are relevant to modern times. The teachings are universal and therefore applicable to all human beings regardless of the country of origin, the religious affiliation, the gender, the age, etc.

Through the practice of the precepts of Maat mental peace and subtlety of intellect (purity of heart) arise. Purity of heart, meaning the absence or anger, hatred, greed, jealousy, discontent, covetousness, elation, stress, agitation, etc. is the means through which divine awareness is possible. When the mind is beset with agitation it is impossible to develop spiritual

The Ancient Egyptian Wisdom Texts

sensitivity. The mind in this state is as if caught in a web of illusion based on the thoughts, desires and ignorance which do not allow awareness of the Divine essence within the heart or in nature, but rather intensify the feelings of individualism, separation and individuality. These in turn open the door for feelings egoistic or personal desires to arise. Feelings of animosity, anger, hatred, greed, jealousy, lust, elation, depression, etc. can only exist when there is individuality or egoism.

Think about it, can you feel jealous of your arm, your head, your foot? No because these are part of you, they are an integral part of your being. In the same way, a perfected (righteous) Sage or Saint sees the entire universe as his or her body and therefore cannot feel jealous, angry, greedy, etc towards anything or anyone. This is because the feeling of ignorance, individuality and separation has been replaced with truth and universality. There is equal vision towards all and universal love for all that exists. This is the experience of an enlightened human being.

The Wisdom texts are to be read, chanted or written daily. This is especially true of the Chapter 125 of Book of Coming Forth By Day. In this manner they are to be studied and practiced so as to engender a mind that is peaceful and harmonious.

The Precepts of Maat and the Philosophy of the Wisdom Texts

> There are two roads traveled by humankind, those who seek to live MAAT, and those who seek to satisfy their animal passions."
>
> —Ancient Egyptian Proverb

The following is a compilation of the 42 laws or precepts of Maat and the corresponding principles which they represent. Maat philosophy was the basis of Ancient Egyptian society and government as well as the heart of Ancient Egyptian myth and spirituality. Maat is at once a goddess, a cosmic force and a living social doctrine, which promotes social harmony and thereby paves the way for spiritual evolution in all levels of society. The Ancient Egyptian Creation myth tells of how God, Ra, created the universe by placing his daughter, Maat, in the place where there was chaos. Maat is the principle of order, harmony, regularity, consistence, peace and truth, which hold the universe together in an orderly fashion. Thus, as a human being that adopts the Maatian lifestyle can come into harmony with the universe (God). Whereas a human being that deviates from Maat will meet with frustration, anxiety, pain and sorrow. In the absence of a social philosophy, which promotes justice, peace and the sublime goals of life, a society cannot function equitably or survive the passage of time. Herein lies the importance of Maat philosophy for the present and future generations.

Other similar social philosophies have developed in other cultures. In India, the philosophy of Dharma, or righteous action, developed. In Christianity the Beatitudes and the new commandments of Jesus serve the same purpose. However, if moral injections are simply memorized but never applied, not understanding their deeper spiritual implications they will not be practiced correctly or at all. Thus the moral character of society declines and strife develops in society. When society places more importance on worldly values and not on spiritual values of life, society declines.

"When opulence and extravagance are a necessity instead of righteousness and truth, society will be governed by greed and injustice."

−Ancient Egyptian Proverb

The injunctions of Maat were statements composed by the Sages of Ancient Egypt and recorded in temple walls and papyrus scrolls, which have survived to this day. They were to be used by spiritual initiates for the purpose of cleansing their personalities and making themselves pure vessels in order to promote spiritual self-discovery. These teachings came to be known as the Book of the Dead. The correct name is Prt m Hru or Pert Em Heru meaning "Utterances for Coming Into the Light of the Most High (Supreme Self-God)" or "The Wisdom and Practices Which Make one Becoming Spiritually Enlightened."

THE 42 INJUNCTIONS OF MAAT AS THEY APPEAR IN THE PERT EM HERU

The following is a composite summary of the "negative confessions" from several Ancient Egyptian Books of Coming Forth by Day. They are often referred to as "Negative Confessions" since the person uttering them is affirming what moral principles they have not transgressed. In this respect they are similar to the Yamas or ethical restraints of India, within the philosophy of Dharma. While all of these books include 42 precepts, some specific precepts varied according to the specific initiate for whom they were prepared and the priests who compiled them. Therefore, I have included more than one precept per line where I felt it was appropriate to show that there were slight variations in the precepts and to more accurately reflect the broader view of the original wisdom imparted by the texts.

The Ancient Egyptian Wisdom Texts

(1) "I have not done iniquity."
   <u>Variant: Acting with falsehood.</u>
(2) "I have not robbed with violence."
(3) "I have not done violence (To anyone or anything)."
   <u>Variant: Rapacious (Taking by force; plundering.)</u>
(4) "I have not committed theft." <u>Variant: Coveted.</u>
(5) "I have not murdered man or woman."
   <u>Variant: Or ordered someone else to commit murder.</u>
(6) "I have not defrauded offerings."
   <u>Variant: or destroyed food supplies or increased or decreased the measures to profit.</u>
(7) "I have not acted deceitfully."
   <u>Variant: With crookedness.</u>
(8) "I have not robbed the things that belong to God."
(9) "I have told no lies."
(10) "I have not snatched away food."
(11) "I have not uttered evil words."
   <u>Variant: Or allowed myself to become sullen, to sulk or become depressed.</u>
(12) "I have attacked no one."
(13) "I have not slaughtered the cattle that are set apart for the Gods."
   <u>Variant: The Sacred bull -Apis)</u>
(14) "I have not eaten my heart" (overcome with anguish and distraught).
   <u>Variant: Committed perjury.</u>
(15) "I have not laid waste the ploughed lands."
(16) "I have not been an eavesdropper or pried into matters to make mischief."
   <u>Variant: Spy.</u>
(17) "I have not spoken against anyone."
   <u>Variant: Babbled, gossiped.</u>
(18) "I have not allowed myself to become angry without cause."
(19) "I have not committed adultery."
   <u>Variant: And homosexuality.</u>
(20) "I have not committed any sin against my own purity."
(21) "I have not violated sacred times and seasons."
(22) "I have not done that which is abominable."
(23) "I have not uttered fiery words. I have not been a man or woman of anger."
(24) "I have not stopped my ears against the words of right and wrong (Maat)."
(25) "I have not stirred up strife (disturbance)." "I have not caused terror." "I have not struck fear into any man."
(26) "I have not caused any one to weep."
   <u>Variant: Hoodwinked.</u>

The Ancient Egyptian Wisdom Texts

(27) "I have not lusted or committed fornication nor have I lain with others of my same sex."
> Variant: or sex with a boy.

(28) "I have not avenged myself."
> Variant: Resentment.

(29) "I have not worked grief, I have not abused anyone."
> Variant: Quarrelsome nature.

(30) "I have not acted insolently or with violence."

(31) "I have not judged hastily."
> Variant: or been impatient.

(32) "I have not transgressed or angered God."

(33) "I have not multiplied my speech overmuch." (Talk too much)

(34) "I have not done harm or evil."
> Variant: Thought evil.

(35) "I have not worked treason or curses on the King."

(36) "I have never befouled the water."
> Variant: held back the water from flowing in its season.

(37) "I have not spoken scornfully."
> Variant: Or yelled unnecessarily or raised my voice.

(38) "I have not cursed The God."

(39) "I have not behaved with arrogance."
> Variant: Boastful.

(40) "I have not been overwhelmingly proud or sought for distinctions for myself (Selfishness)."

(41) "I have never magnified my condition beyond what was fitting or increased my wealth, except with such things as are (justly) mine own possessions by means of Maat."
> Variant: I have not disputed over possessions except when they concern my own rightful possessions. Variant: I have not desired more than what is rightfully mine.

(42) "I have never thought evil (blasphemed) or slighted The God in my native town."

The Ancient Egyptian Wisdom Texts

THE DISCIPLINE AND PHILOSOPHY OF RIGHTEOUS ACTION

> "The wise person who acts with MAAT is free of falsehood and disorder."
>
> -Ancient Egyptian Proverb

The teachings of Pert em Heru are related to the Yoga of Righteous Action. The word Yoga originates in the Indian Sanskrit, meaning union of the lower self (mortal personality) with the higher(immortal spiritual Self). Since there is no direct translation for Yoga in the English language and since it has been assimilated into the English language, it will be used as the English translation of the word interchangeably with the Indian Sanskrit term as well as the Ancient Egyptian term. In Ancient Egypt the main word-symbol for Yoga was Smai. Yoga is the practice of spiritual disciplines, a way of life, which lead to positive spiritual evolution. There are four major aspects of Yoga: The Yoga of Wisdom, The Yoga of Devotion, The Yoga of Meditation and the Yoga of Righteous Action.

The teachings of righteous action originated in the early history of Ancient Egypt with the writings of the Ancient Egyptian Sages, known as the "Wisdom Texts." There were many Sages in Ancient Egypt, however, only a relatively small number of their writings have survived. Nevertheless, these are enough to provide a viable understanding of the Ancient Egyptian wisdom teachings and these writings reveal the source of the Maatian precepts and philosophy contained in the Pert em Heru. Therefore, as we study the precepts of Maat, along with the Wisdom Texts, we will obtain a deeper insight into the profound nature of the precepts.

The Sages of ancient times noticed that action is the inescapable fact of life. Everyone must be engaged in one form of action or another. However, if one's actions are based on ignorance and egoism then they lead to unnecessary entanglements and negative situations in life that ultimately cause pain and sorrow (Negative Karma). The Sages then set out to develop a system of philosophy which will lead a person to act correctly in life and discover the inner reaches of their own higher self. The practice and perfection of action affords a human being the

The Ancient Egyptian Wisdom Texts

opportunity to purify his or her heart. This leads to a life of peace, harmony with nature and society and ultimately to spiritual enlightenment as well (Positive Karma). The teaching of Karma is embodied in the following Ancient Egyptian teaching from the Instructions of Merikara:

> (14) The Court that judges the wretch,
> You know they are not lenient,
> On the day of judging the miserable,
> In the hour of doing their task.
> It is painful when the accuser has knowledge,
> Do not trust in length of years,
> They view a lifetime in an hour!
> When a man remains over after death,
> His deeds are set beside him as treasure,
> And being yonder lasts forever.
> A fool is who does what they reprove!
> He who reaches them without having done wrong
>
> Will exist there like a god,
> Free-striding like the lords forever!

Karma is a Sanskrit word which has been assimilated into the English language. The Ancient Egyptian term is Meskhenet. Meskhenet is the accumulated sum total of a person's mental impression which they gathered through their past feelings, desires, and beliefs, based on their previous actions. They are impressions stored in the mind, which impel a person to actions in accordance with the nature of the impressions. There is no equivalent word in the English language for Karma but this Indian word has been assimilated into Western culture. The Ancient Egyptian term for Karma is Meskhenet. Karma is not destiny or fate. It can be changed in accordance with a person's present actions and new understanding. So a person can change a bad situation into a good situation and spiritual ignorance and degradation into spiritual enlightenment by changing the actions in life from unrighteous to righteous, from those based on spiritual ignorance to those based on spiritual wisdom.

The numbers of each precept denotes the order in which it appears in the Papyrus of Ani or Pertem heru of Initiate Ani. Since there are various

The Ancient Egyptian Wisdom Texts

Pert em Herus which have been discovered and no two have the same exact wording, variants will also be included to elucidate on the expanded meanings accorded to the precepts of different Sages as recorded by the scribes.

The 42 precepts may be classified into six major principles and within these more can be subdivided. The six principles are Truthfulness, Non-violence, Right Action, Right Thinking, Non-stealing and Sex Sublimation. The subdivisions are under Right Action. They are Selfless Service to Humanity, Right Speech and Right Worship of the Divine or Correct Spiritual Practice.

Truth (1), (6), (7), (9), (24)
Non-violence (2), (3), (5), (12), (25), (26), (28), (30), (34)
Non-stealing (4), (8), (10)
Self-Control-Right Action (Living in accordance with the teachings of Maat) (15), (20), (22), (36)
    Selfless Service, (29)
    Right Speech (11), (17), (23), (33), (35), (37)
    Right Worship (13), (21), (32), (38), (42)
Balance of Mind - Reason - Right Thinking (14), (16), (18), (31), (39), (41)
    Sex-Sublimation (19), (27)

The Ancient Egyptian Wisdom Texts

What is a Sage?

'*(He is the one) whose heart is informed about these things which would be otherwise ignored, the one who is clear-sighted when he is deep into a problem, the one who is moderate in his actions, who penetrates ancient writings, who is sensible enough to unravel complications, who is really wise, who instructed his own heart, who stays awake at night as he looks for the right paths, who surpasses what he accomplished yesterday, who is wiser than a sage, who brought himself to wisdom, who asks for advice and sees to it that he is asked for advice*'

(*Inscription of an Antef,* 12th dynasty: Middle Kingdom, I 11th and 12th dynasties, 2052 -1778 B.C.E.)
translated by the German Egyptologist Hellmut Brunner:

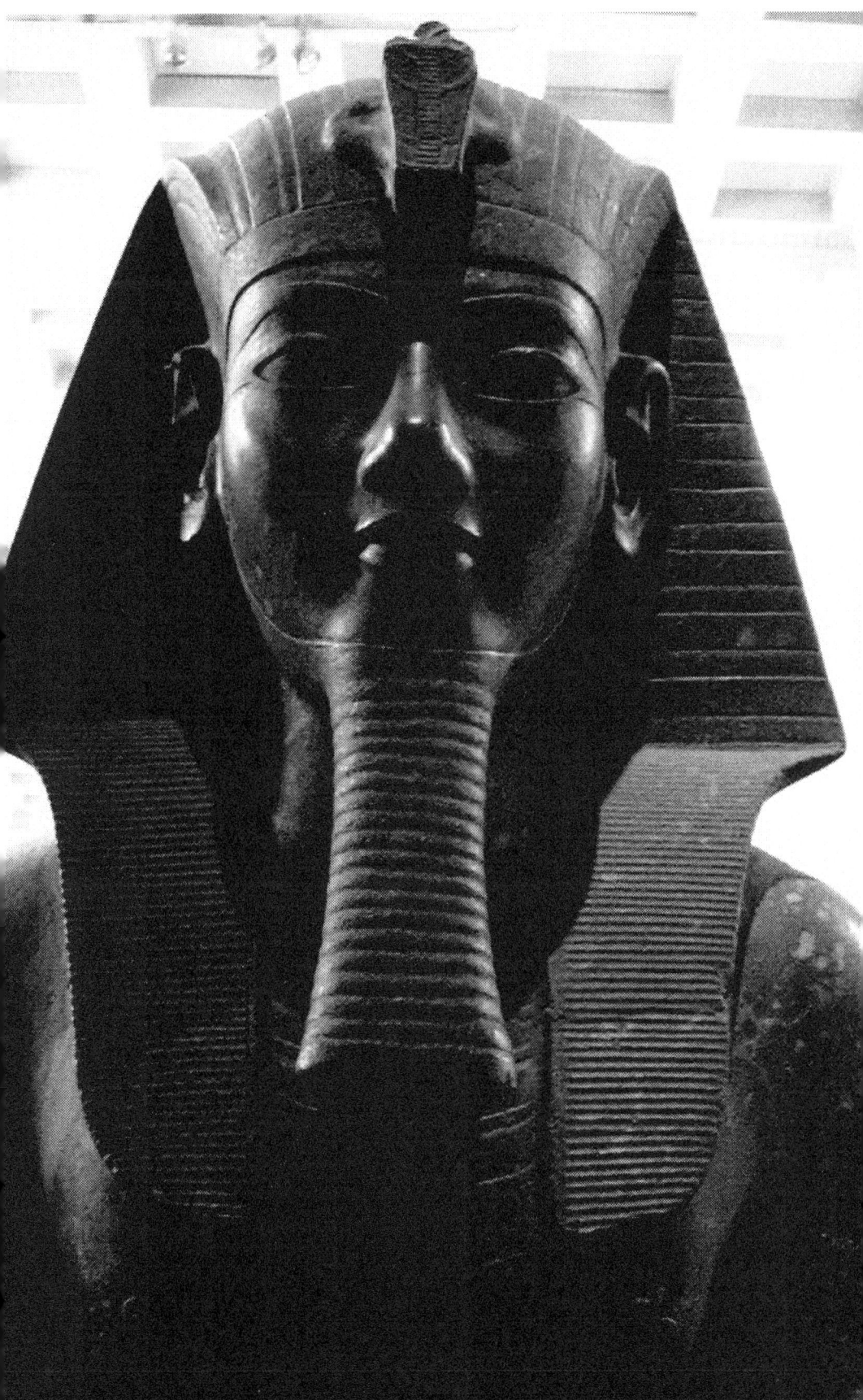

The Ancient Egyptian Wisdom Texts

The Teachings of Ptahotep

The Instruction of the Governor of his City, the Vizier, Ptah-hotep, in the Reign of the King of Upper and Lower Egypt, Isôsi, living for ever, to the end of Time.

A. The Governor of his City, the Vizier, Ptah-hotep, he said: 'O Prince, my Lord, the end of life is at hand; old age descendeth [upon me]; feebleness cometh, and childishness is renewed. He [that is old] lieth down in misery every day. The eyes are small; the ears are deaf. Energy is diminished, the heart hath no rest. The mouth is silent, and he speaketh no word; the heart stoppeth, and he remembereth not yesterday. The bones are painful throughout the body; good turneth unto evil. All taste departeth. These things doeth old age for mankind, being evil in all things. The nose is stopped, and he breatheth not for weakness (?), whether standing or sitting.

'Command me, thy servant, therefore, to make over my princely authority [to my son]. Let me speak unto him the words of them that hearken to the counsel of the men of old time; those that hearkened unto the gods. I pray thee, let this thing be done, that sin may be banished from among persons of understanding, that thou may enlighten the lands.'

Said the Majesty of this God :[1] 'Instruct him, then, in the words of old time ; may he be a wonder unto the children of princes, that they may enter and hearken with him. Make straight all their hearts ; and discourse with him, without causing weariness.'

B. Here begin the proverbs of fair speech, spoken by the Hereditary Chief, the Holy Father,[2] Beloved of the God, the Eldest Son of the King, of his body, the Governor of his City, the Vezier, Ptah-hotep, when instructing the ignorant in the knowledge of exactness in fair-speaking ; the glory of him that obeyeth, the shame of him that transgresseth them.

He said unto his son :

1. Be not proud because thou art learned ; but discourse with the ignorant man, as with the sage. For no limit can be set to skill, neither is there any craftsman that possesseth full advantages. Fair speech is more rare than the emerald that is found by slave-maidens on the pebbles.

2. If thou find an arguer talking, one that is well disposed and wiser than thou, let thine arms

---

[1] The King.   [2] Title of an order of the priesthood.

fall, bend thy back,[1] be not angry with him if he agree (?) not with thee. Refrain from speaking evilly; oppose him not at any time when he speaketh. If he address thee as one ignorant of the matter, thine humbleness shall bear away his contentions.

3. If thou find an arguer talking, thy fellow, one that is within thy reach, keep not silence when he saith aught that is evil; so shalt thou be wiser than he. Great will be the applause on the part of the listeners, and thy name shall be good in the knowledge of princes.

4. If thou find an arguer talking, a poor man, that is to say not thine equal, be not scornful toward him because he is lowly. Let him alone; then shall he confound himself. Question him not to please thine heart, neither pour out thy wrath upon him that is before thee; it is shameful to confuse a mean mind. If thou be about to do that which is in thine heart, overcome it as a thing rejected of princes.

5. If thou be a leader, as one directing the conduct of the multitude, endeavour always to be gracious, that thine own conduct be without defect. Great is Truth, appointing a straight path; never hath it been overthrown since the

[1] The customary attitude of a submissive inferior at that time.

reign of Osiris.¹ One that oversteppeth the laws shall be punished. Overstepping is by the covetous man; but degradations (?) bear off his riches, for the season of his evil-doing ceaseth not. For he saith, 'I will obtain by myself for myself,' and saith not, 'I will obtain because I am allowed.' But the limits of justice are steadfast; it is that which a man repeateth from his father.

6. Cause not fear among men; for [this] the God punisheth likewise. For there is a man that saith, 'Therein is life'; and he is bereft of the bread of his mouth. There is a man that saith, 'Power [is therein]'; and he saith, 'I seize for myself that which I perceive.' Thus a man speaketh, and he is smitten down. It is another that attaineth by giving unto him that hath not; not he that causeth men dread. For it happeneth that what the God hath commanded, even that thing cometh to pass. Live, therefore, in the house of kindliness, and men shall come and give gifts of themselves.

7. If thou be among the guests of a man that is greater than thou, accept that which he giveth thee, putting it to thy lips. If thou look at him that is before thee (thine host), pierce him not

¹ The God Osiris was believed to have reigned on earth many thousand years before Mênês, the first historical king.

The Ancient Egyptian Wisdom Texts

with many glances. It is abhorred of the soul [1] to stare at him. Speak not till he address thee; one knoweth not what may be evil in his opinion. Speak when he questioneth thee; so shall thy speech be good in his opinion. The noble who sitteth before food divideth it as his soul moveth him; he giveth unto him that he would favour—it is the custom of the evening meal. It is his soul that guideth his hand. It is the noble that bestoweth, not the underling that attaineth. Thus the eating of bread is under the providence of the God; he is an ignorant man that disputeth it.

8. If thou be an emissary sent from one noble to another, be exact after the manner of him that sent thee, give his message even as he hath said it. Beware of making enmity by thy words, setting one noble against the other by perverting truth. Overstep it not, neither repeat that which any man, be he prince or peasant, saith in opening the heart; it is abhorrent to the soul.

9. If thou have ploughed, gather thine harvest in the field, and the God shall make it great under thine hand. Fill not thy mouth at thy neighbours' table. . . . [2] If a crafty man be the

---

[1] Soul = *ka'*, and throughout this work. *Ka'* is translated *person* in § 22, *will* in § 27.

[2] An obscure or corrupt phrase here follows, which does not admit of satisfactory translation.

The Ancient Egyptian Wisdom Texts

possessor of wealth, he stealeth like a crocodile from the priests.

Let not a man be envious that hath no children; let him be neither downcast nor quarrelsome on account of it. For a father, though great, may be grieved; as to the mother of children, she hath less peace than another. Verily, each man is created [to his destiny] by the God, Who is the chief of a tribe, trustful in following him.

10. If thou be lowly, serve a wise man, that all thine actions may be good before the God. If thou have known a man of none account that hath been advanced in rank, be not haughty toward him on account of that which thou knowest concerning him; but honour him that hath been advanced, according to that which he hath become.

Behold, riches come not of themselves; it is their rule for him that desireth them. If he bestir him and collect them himself, the God shall make him prosperous; but He shall punish him, if he be slothful.

11. Follow thine heart during thy lifetime; do not more than is commanded thee. Diminish not the time of following the heart; it is abhorred of the soul, that its time [of ease] be taken away. Shorten not the daytime more than is needful to

FROM FATHER TO SON

maintain thine house. When riches are gained, follow the heart; for riches are of no avail if one be weary.

12. If thou wouldest be a wise man, beget a son for the pleasing of the God. If he make straight his course after thine example, if he arrange thine affairs in due order, do unto him all that is good, for thy son is he, begotten of thine own soul. Sunder not thine heart from him, or thine own begotten shall curse [thee]. If he be heedless and trespass thy rules of conduct, and is violent; if every speech that cometh from his mouth be a vile word; then beat thou him, that his talk may be fitting. Keep him from those that make light of that which is commanded, for it is they that make him rebellious.[1] And they that are guided go not astray, but they that lose their bearings cannot find a straight course.

13. If thou be in the chamber of council, act always according to the steps enjoined on thee at the beginning of the day. Be not absent, or thou shalt be expelled; but be ready in entering and making report. Wide[2] is the seat of one that hath made address. The council-chamber acteth by strict rule; and all its plans are in accordance with method. It is the God that

[1] Translation doubtful.   [2] *i.e.* comfortable.

advanceth one to a seat therein; the like is not done for elbowers.

14. If thou be among people, make for thyself love, the beginning and end of the heart. One that knoweth not his course shall say in himself (seeing thee), 'He that ordereth himself duly becometh the owner of wealth; I shall copy his conduct.' Thy name shall be good, though thou speak not; thy body shall be fed; thy face shall be [seen] among thy neighbours; thou shalt be provided with what thou lackest. As to the man whose heart obeyeth his belly, he causeth disgust in place of love. His heart is wretched (?), his body is gross (?), he is insolent toward those endowed of the God. He that obeyeth his belly hath an enemy.[1]

15. Report thine actions without concealment; discover thy conduct when in council with thine overlord. It is not evil for the envoy that his report be not answered, 'Yea, I know it,' by the prince; for that which he knoweth includeth not [this]. If he (the prince) think that he will oppose him on account of it, [he thinketh] 'He will be silent because I have spoken.'[2]

16. If thou be a leader, cause that the rules

[1] His belly, presumably.
[2] The above translation is not satisfactory; the text may be corrupt. No intelligible translation of it has yet been made.

A JUST JUDGE

that thou hast enjoined be carried out; and do all things as one that remembereth the days coming after, when speech availeth not. Be not lavish of favours; it leadeth to servility (?), producing slackness.

17. If thou be a leader, be gracious when thou hearkenest unto the speech of a suppliant. Let him not hesitate to deliver himself of that which he hath thought to tell thee; but be desirous of removing his injury. Let him speak freely, that the thing for which he hath come to thee may be done. If he hesitate to open his heart, it is said, 'Is it because he (the judge) doeth the wrong that no entreaties are made to him concerning it by those to whom it happeneth?' But a well-taught heart hearkeneth readily.

18. If thou desire to continue friendship in any abode wherein thou enterest, be it as master, as brother, or as friend; wheresoever thou goest, beware of consorting with women. No place prospereth wherein that is done. Nor is it prudent to take part in it; a thousand men have been ruined for the pleasure of a little time short as a dream. Even death is reached thereby; it is a wretched thing. As for the evil liver, one leaveth him for what he doeth, he is avoided. If his desires be not gratified, he regardeth (?) no laws.

19. If thou desire that thine actions may be good, save thyself from all malice, and beware of the quality of covetousness, which is a grievous inner (?) malady. Let it not chance that thou fall thereinto. It setteth at variance fathers-in-law and the kinsmen of the daughter-in-law; it sundereth the wife and the husband. It gathereth unto itself all evils; it is the girdle of all wickedness.[1] But the man that is just flourisheth; truth goeth in his footsteps, and he maketh habitations therein, not in the dwelling of covetousness.

20. Be not covetous as touching shares, in seizing that which is not thine own property. Be not covetous toward thy neighbours; for with a gentle man praise availeth more than might. He [that is covetous] cometh empty from among his neighbours, being void of the persuasion of speech. One hath remorse for even a little covetousness when his belly cooleth.

21. If thou wouldest be wise, provide for thine house, and love thy wife that is in thine arms. Fill her stomach, clothe her back; oil is the remedy of her limbs. Gladden her heart during thy lifetime, for she is an estate profitable unto its lord. Be not harsh, for gentleness mastereth her more than strength. Give (?) to her that for which she sigheth and that toward which her

---

[1] *i.e.* all wickedness is contained therein.

THE TREATMENT OF SERVANTS

eye looketh; so shalt thou keep her in thine house. . . .

22. Satisfy thine hired servants out of such things as thou hast; it is the duty of one that hath been favoured of the God. In sooth, it is hard to satisfy hired servants. For one [1] saith, 'He is a lavish person; one knoweth not that which may come [from him].' But on the morrow he thinketh, 'He is a person of exactitude (parsimony), content therein.' And when favours have been shown unto servants, they say, 'We go.' Peace dwelleth not in that town wherein dwell servants that are wretched.

23. Repeat not extravagant speech, neither listen thereto; for it is the utterance of a body heated by wrath. When such speech is repeated to thee, hearken not thereto, look to the ground. Speak not regarding it, that he that is before thee may know wisdom. If thou be commanded to do a theft, bring it to pass that the command be taken off thee, for it is a thing hateful according to law. That which destroyeth a vision is the veil over it.

24. If thou wouldest be a wise man, and one sitting in council with his overlord, apply thine heart unto perfection. Silence is more profitable unto thee than abundance of speech. Consider

[1] A servant.

how thou may be opposed by an expert that speaketh in council. It is a foolish thing to speak on every kind of work, for he that disputeth thy words shall put them unto proof.

25. If thou be powerful, make thyself to be honoured for knowledge and for gentleness. Speak with authority, that is, not as if following injunctions, for he that is humble (when highly placed) falleth into errors. Exalt not thine heart, that it be not brought low.[1] Be not silent, but beware of interruption and of answering words with heat. Put it far from thee; control thyself. The wrathful heart speaketh fiery words; it darteth out at the man of peace that approacheth, stopping his path.

One that reckoneth accounts all the day passeth not an happy moment. One that gladdeneth his heart all the day provideth not for his house. The bowman hitteth the mark, as the steersman reacheth land, by diversity of aim. He that obeyeth his heart shall command.[2]

26. Let not a prince be hindered when he is occupied; neither oppress the heart of him that is already laden. For he shall be hostile toward one that delayeth him, but shall bare his soul

[1] Compare Prov. xvii. 18.
[2] So also in life, by diversity of aim, alternating work and play, happiness is secured. Tacking is evidently meant in the case of the steersman.

DUTIES OF THE GREAT

unto one that loveth him. The disposal of souls is with the God, and that which He loveth is His creation. Set out, therefore, after a violent quarrel; be at peace with him that is hostile unto [thee] his opponent. It is such souls that make love to grow.

27. Instruct a noble in such things as be profitable unto him; cause that he be received among men. Let his satisfaction fall on his master, for thy provision dependeth upon his will. By reason of it thy belly shall be satisfied; thy back will be clothed thereby. Let him receive thine heart, that thine house may flourish and thine honour—if thou wish it to flourish—thereby. He shall extend thee a kindly hand. Further, he shall implant the love of thee in the bodies of thy friends. Forsooth, it is a soul loving to hearken.[1]

28. If thou be the son of a man of the priesthood, and an envoy to conciliate the multitude, ...[2] speak thou without favouring one side. Let it not be said, 'His conduct is that of the nobles, favouring one side in his speech.' Turn thine aim toward exact judgments.

---

[1] This section refers to the relations between the son of a nobleman and his tutor, dwelling on the benefits from former pupils in high places, if their schooldays have been pleasant. The last sentence of this section, as of sections 23 and 25, is somewhat *à propos des bottes*.

[2] An obscure phrase is here.

29. If thou have been gracious at a former time, having forgiven a man to guide him aright, shun him, remind him not after the first day that he hath been silent to thee [concerning it].

30. If thou be great, after being of none account, and hast gotten riches after squalor, being foremost in these in the city, and hast knowledge concerning useful matters, so that promotion is come unto thee; then swathe not thine heart in thine hoard, for thou art become the steward of the endowments of the God. Thou art not the last; another shall be thine equal, and to him shall come the like [fortune and station].

31. Bend thy back unto thy chief, thine overseer in the King's palace, for thine house dependeth upon his wealth, and thy wages in their season. How foolish is one that quarrelleth with his chief, for one liveth only while he is gracious. . . .

Plunder not the houses of tenants; neither steal the things of a friend, lest he accuse thee in thine hearing, which thrusteth back the heart.[1] If he know of it, he will do thee an injury. Quarrelling in place of friendship is a foolish thing.

[1] Literally, "It is that which preventeth the heart from advancing (?)" A curious phrase.

THE TEST OF FRIENDSHIP

32. [Concerning continence].

33. If thou wouldest seek out the nature of a friend, ask it not of any companion of his; but pass a time with him alone, that thou injure not his affairs. Debate with him after a season; test his heart in an occasion of speech. When he hath told thee his past life, he hath made an opportunity that thou may either be ashamed for him or be familiar with him. Be not reserved with him when he openeth speech, neither answer him after a scornful manner. Withdraw not thyself from him, neither interrupt (?) him whose matter is not yet ended, whom it is possible to benefit.

34. Let thy face be bright what time thou livest. That which goeth into the storehouse must come out therefrom; and bread is to be shared. He that is grasping in entertainment shall himself have an empty belly; he that causeth strife cometh himself to sorrow. Take not such an one for thy companion. It is a man's kindly acts that are remembered of him in the years after his life.[1]

35. Know well thy merchants; for when thine affairs are in evil case, thy good repute among thy friends is a channel (?) which is filled. It is more important than the dignities of a man; and

[1] Literally, after his stick or sceptre.

the wealth of one passeth to another. The good repute of a man's son is a glory unto him; and a good character is for remembrance.

36. Correct chiefly; instruct conformably [therewith]. Vice must be drawn out, that virtue may remain. Nor is this a matter of misfortune, for one that is a gainsayer becometh a strife-maker.

37. If thou make a woman to be ashamed, wanton of heart, one known by her townsfolk to be falsely placed, be kind unto her for a space, send her not away, give her to eat. The wantonness of her heart shall esteem thy guidance.

C. If thou obey these things that I have said unto thee, all thy demeanour shall be of the best; for, verily, the quality of truth is among their excellences. Set the memory of them in the mouths of the people; for their proverbs are good. Nor shall any word that hath here been set down cease out of this land for ever, but shall be made a pattern whereby princes shall speak well. They (my words) shall instruct a man how he shall speak, after he hath heard them; yea, he shall become as one skilful in obeying, excellent in speaking, after he hath heard them. Good fortune shall befall him, for he shall be of the highest rank. He shall be gracious to the end of his life; he shall be con-

THE BEAUTY OF OBEDIENCE

tented always. His knowledge shall be his guide (?) into a place of security, wherein he shall prosper while on earth. The scholar [1] shall be content in his knowledge. As to the prince, in his turn, forsooth, his heart shall be happy, his tongue made straight. And [in these proverbs] his lips shall speak, his eyes shall see, and his ears shall hear, that which is profitable for his son, so that he deal justly, void of deceit.

38. A splendid thing is the obedience of an obedient son; he cometh in and listeneth obediently.

Excellent in hearing, excellent in speaking, is every man that obeyeth what is noble; and the obedience of an obeyer is a noble thing.

Obedience is better than all things that are; it maketh good-will.

How good it is that a son should take that from his father by which he hath reached old age (Obedience).

That which is desired by the God is obedience; disobedience is abhorred of the God.

Verily, it is the heart that maketh its master to obey or to disobey; for the safe and sound life of a man are his heart.

It is the obedient man that obeyeth what is said; he that loveth to obey, the same shall carry out commands.

[1] Who knows them.

He that obeyeth becometh one obeyed.

It is good indeed when a son obeyeth his father; and he (his father) that hath spoken hath great joy of it. Such a son shall be mild as a master, and he that heareth him shall obey him that hath spoken. He shall be comely in body and honoured by his father. His memory shall be in the mouths of the living, those upon earth, as long as they exist.[1]

39. Let a son receive the word of his father, not being heedless of any rule of his. Instruct thy son [thus]; for the obedient man is one that is perfect in the opinion of princes. If he direct his mouth by what hath been enjoined him, watchful and obedient, thy son shall be wise, and his goings seemly. Heedlessness leadeth unto disobedience on the morrow; but understanding shall stablish him. As for the fool, he shall be crushed.

40. As for the fool, devoid of obedience, he doeth nothing. Knowledge he regardeth as ignorance, profitable things as hurtful things. He doeth all kind of errors, so that he is rebuked therefor every day. He liveth in death there-

---

[1] The greater part of this section is a play upon the root *śôdem*, which in its meaning includes our *hear* (*listen*) and *obey*. This tiresome torture of words is frequent in Egyptian, especially in old religious texts.

ONE GENERATION TO ANOTHER

with; it is his food. At chattering speech he marvelleth, as at the wisdom of princes, living in death every day. He is shunned because of his misfortunes, by reason of the multitude of afflictions that cometh upon him every day.

41. A son that hearkeneth is as a Follower of Horus.[1] He is good after he hearkeneth; he groweth old, he reacheth honour and reverence. He repeateth in like manner to his sons and daughters, so renewing the instruction of his father. Each man instructeth as did his begetter, repeating it unto his children. Let them [in turn] speak with their sons and daughters, that they may be famous in their deeds. Let that which thou speakest implant true things and just in the life of thy children. Then the highest authority shall arrive, and sins depart [from them]. And such men as see these things shall say, 'Surely that man hath spoken to good purpose,' and they shall do likewise; or, 'But surely that man was experienced.' And all people shall declare, 'It is they that shall direct the multitude; dignities are not complete without them.'

Take not any word away, neither add one;

[1] The "Followers of Horus" are a legendary dynasty of demigods, believed by the Egyptians to have ruled for about 13,400 years after the reign of Horus, and before that of Mênês. There is also an order of spirits of this name.

set not one in the place of another. Beware of opening . . .[1] in thyself.

Be wary of speech when a learned man hearkeneth unto thee; desire to be stablished for good in the mouth of those that hear thee speaking. If thou have entered as an expert, speak with exact (?) lips, that thy conduct may be seemly.

42. Be thine heart overflowing; but refrain thy mouth. Let thy conduct be exact while amongst nobles, and seemly before thy lord, doing that which he hath commanded. Such a son shall speak unto them that hearken to him; moreover, his begetter shall be favoured. Apply thine heart, what time thou speakest, to saying things such that the nobles who listen declare, 'How excellent is that which cometh out of his mouth!'

43. Carry out the behest of thy lord to thee. How good is the teaching of a man's father, for he hath come from him, who hath spoken of his son while he was yet unborn; and that which is done for him (the son) is more than that which is commanded him. Forsooth, a good son is of the gift of the God; he doeth more than is

---

[1] A word of unknown meaning; apparently some kind of plant. Such a word seems out of place here, and may be idiomatic, like our "flowery language." But the preceding line obviously refers to this book.

WHOM THE KING HONOURETH

enjoined on him, he doeth right, and putteth his heart into all his goings.

D. If now thou attain my position, thy body shall flourish, the King shall be content in all that thou doest, and thou shalt gather years of life not fewer than I have passed upon earth. I have gathered even fivescore and ten years of life, for the King hath bestowed upon me favours more than upon my forefathers; this because I wrought truth and justice for the King unto mine old age.

**IT IS FINISHED
FROM ITS BEGINNING TO ITS END
EVEN AS FOUND IN WRITING.**

The Ancient Egyptian Wisdom Texts

The Teachings of Kagemni

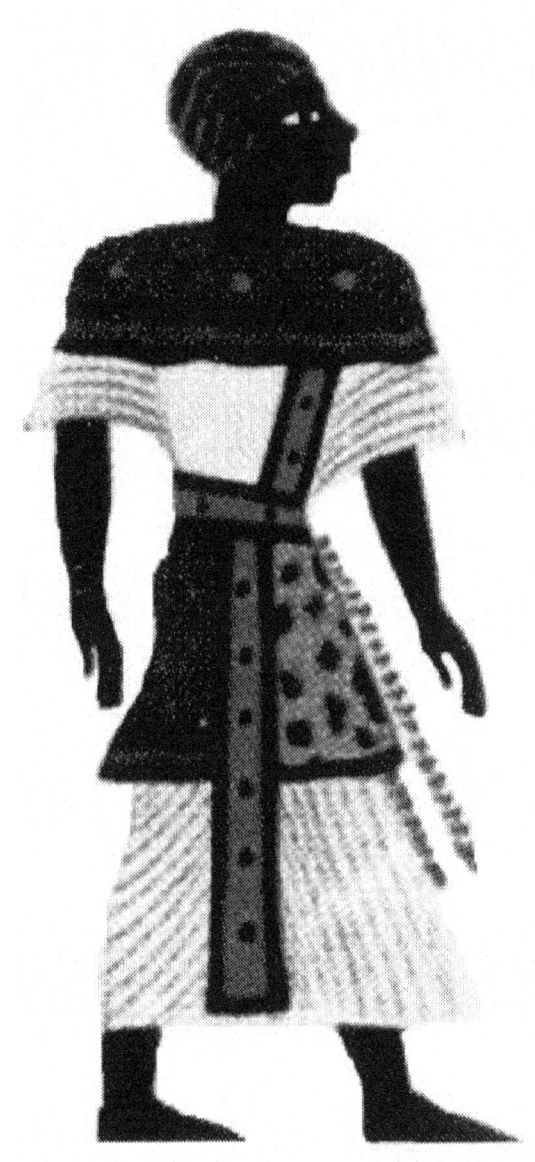

The Ancient Egyptian Wisdom Texts

1.[1] The cautious man flourisheth, the exact one is praised; the innermost chamber openeth unto the man of silence. Wide [2] is the seat of the man gentle of speech; but knives are prepared against one that forceth a path, that he advance not, save in due season.

2. If thou sit with a company of people, desire not the bread that thou likest: short is the time of restraining the heart, and gluttony is an abomination; therein is the quality of a beast. A cup of water quencheth the thirst, and a mouthful of melon supporteth the heart. A good thing standeth for goodness, but some small thing standeth for plenty.[3] A base man is he that is governed by his belly; he departeth only when he is no longer able to fill full his belly in men's houses.

---

[1] The original is not divided into sections.

[2] *i.e.* comfortable

[3] This is a rather dark saying, but apparently the author means that although the duly instructed guest will only partake moderately of the abundance before him, what he eats is as good as the rest. His portion will be equal to the whole as regards quality, though inferior as regards quantity.

ON AVOIDING OFFENCE

3. If thou sit with a glutton, eat with him, then depart (?).

If thou drink with a drunkard, accept [drink], and his heart shall be satisfied.

Refuse not meat when with a greedy man. Take that which he giveth thee; set it not on one side, thinking that it will be a courteous thing.

4. If a man be lacking in good fellowship, no speech hath any influence over him. He is sour of face toward the glad-hearted that are kindly to him; he is a grief unto his mother and his friends; and all men [cry], ' Let thy name be known; thou art silent in thy mouth when thou art addressed ! '

5. Be not haughty because of thy might in the midst of thy young soldiers. Beware of making strife, for one knoweth not the things that the God will do when He punisheth.

The Vizier caused his sons and daughters to be summoned, when he had finished the rules of the conduct of men. And they marvelled when they came to him. Then he said unto them, ' Hearken unto everything that is in writing in this book, even as I have said it in adding unto profitable sayings.' And they cast themselves on their bellies, and they read it, even as it was in writing. And it was better in their opinion than any thing in this land unto its limits.

Now they were living when His Majesty, the King of Upper and Lower Egypt, Heuni, departed, and His Majesty, the King of Upper and Lower Egypt, Senfôru, was enthroned as a gracious king over the whole of this land.

Then was Ke'gemni made Governor of his City and Vizier.

IT IS FINISHED.

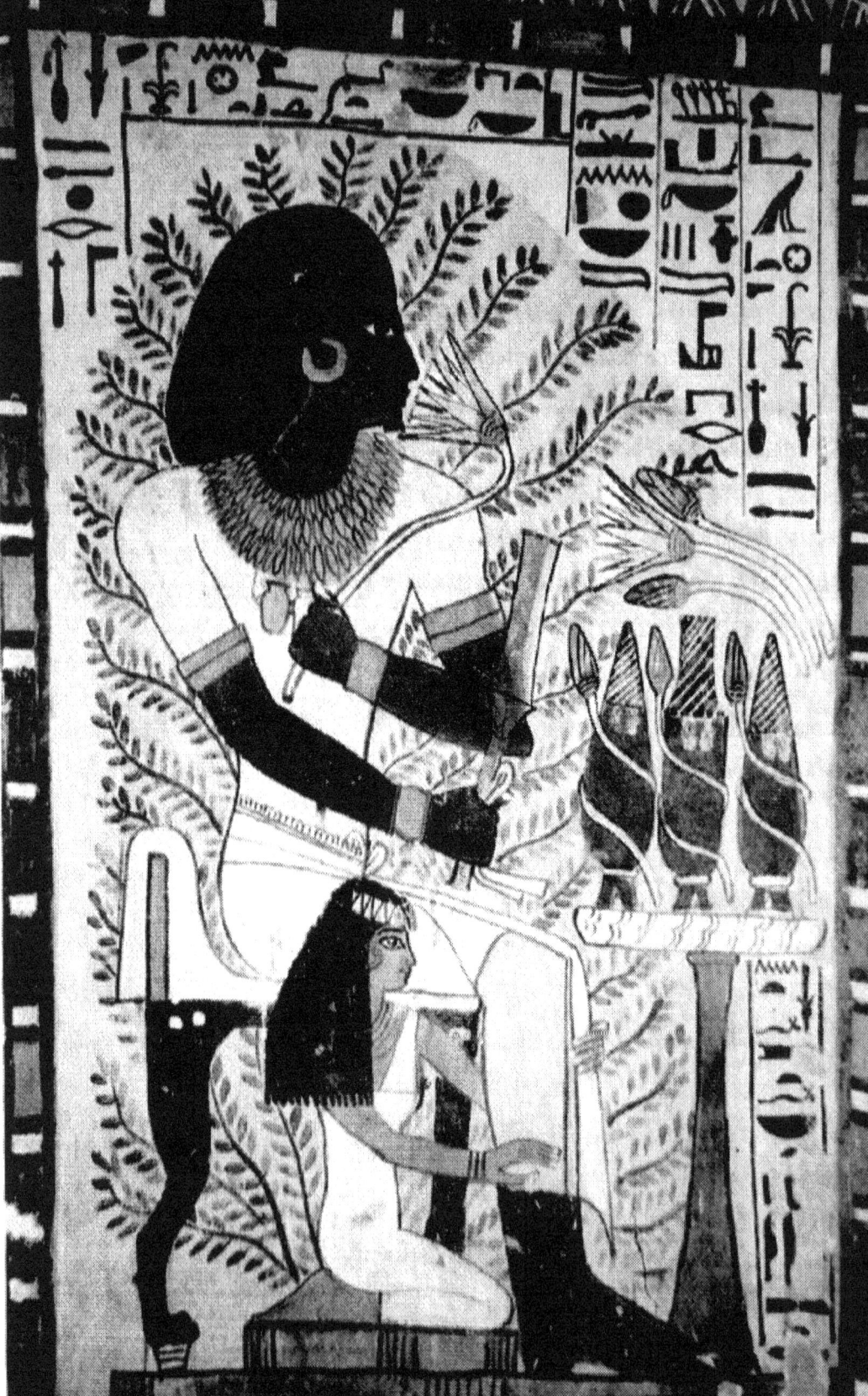

The Ancient Egyptian Wisdom Texts

The Teachings of Amunemhat

This book also seems to have been held in high esteem during the New Kingdom, for it is preserved in four different papyri, and extracts from it are found on at least nine ostraca. Unfortunately there is no older manuscript, and, with one exception, they are all writing-exercises of schoolboys of the Nineteenth Dynasty (*circa* 1300 B.C.), and teem with mistakes.

The great king Amenemhēt I (1955–1965 B.C.), in the twentieth year of his reign, as we know from other sources, made his son Sesōstris I co-regent, and withdrew from the outward activities of political life.

Our document represents the aged king as recounting to his son on this occasion, by way of admonishment, the events which induced him to take this step; he had reaped ingratitude, and an attempt had been made on his life.

Instruction, which the majesty of King Sehetepibrē,[2] the son of Rē, Amenemhēt, made, speaking in a message of truth to his son, the Lord of All.

He saith: "Thou that hast appeared as God,[3] hearken to what I shall say to thee, that thou mayest be king over the land, and ruler over the river banks, that thou mayest do good in excess of (what is looked for). Be on thy guard against subordinates – – – –; approach them not, and be not alone. Trust not a brother, know not a friend, and make not for thyself intimates,—that profiteth nothing.

If thou sleepest, do thou thyself guard thine heart, for in the day of adversity a man hath no adherents. I gave to the poor and nourished the orphan, I caused him that was nothing to reach the goal, even as him that was of account.

It was he who ate my food that disdained me (?); it was he to whom I gave my hand that aroused fear therewith.[4] They that clothed them in my fine linen looked at me as at a

---

[1] See the article by GRIFFITH in *Zeitschr. für ägypt. Sprache*, xxxiv. pp. 35 ff.; MASPERO, *Les ensignements d'Amenemhâit I*er*. Cairo, 1914.

[2] "He who pacifies the heart of Rē," the official name of King Amenemhēt I.

[3] *I.e.* that hast become king.

[4] With the kindness which I showed him?

The Ancient Egyptian Wisdom Texts

shadow, and they that anointed them with my myrrh, poured water . . .

Mine images are among the living, and my shares (in the offerings) among men;[1] (and yet?) they contrived a conspiracy (?) against me, without it being heard, and a great contest, without it being seen.[2] Men fought on the place of combat[3] and forgat yesterday.[4]—Good fortune attendeth not one that knoweth not when he ought (?) to know.[5]

It was after supper, when night had come; I had taken an hour of repose, and laid me down upon my bed. I was weary, and my heart began to follow after slumber. Then it was as if weapons were brandished, and as if one inquired (?) concerning me, and I became like a snake of the desert.[6]

I roused me, to fight alone (?), and I marked that it was an hand-to-hand affray of the bodyguard. When I had quickly taken weapons into mine hand, I drave back the rogues. . . . But there is no strength by night, and one cannot (?) fight alone, and success will not come without thee that protectest me.[7]

Behold, the abominable thing came to pass when I was without thee, when the Court had not yet heard that I am resigning (the sovereign power) to thee,[8] when I did not yet dwell with thee. May I act according to thy counsels,[9] for I fear them[10] no (more), . . . *and I am powerless against* the indolence of servants.

Had the women set the battle in array? Had the conflict been fostered (?) within the house? — — — — Were the townsmen made foolish on account of their[11] deeds. Ill fortune hath not come behind me since my birth, and nought hath happened that might equal my prowess as a doer of valiant deeds.[12]

---

[1] So honoured am I in the land.
[2] No one betrayed to me the plot.
[3] Literally the place where the bulls fight. [4] My good deeds.
[5] Does he mean himself, who was unsuspicious? The interpretation of the whole paragraph is by no means certain. (See also GUNN, *Syntax*, p. 128 [Translator]).
[6] *I.e.* I started up like a sand-viper.
[7] He fears further assaults if his son is not associated with him on the throne.
[8] That sounds as though the attempt had been made by some one who wished to see the son on the throne at once.
[9] *I.e.* your plan to take a part in governing.
[10] The courtiers. [11] The conspirators?
[12] For this successful administration I have had but ill thanks.

The Ancient Egyptian Wisdom Texts

I trod Elephantine,[1] I marched into the Delta; I stood upon the boundaries of the land and beheld its circuit. I carried forward the boundaries of my power by my might and by my prowess.

I was one that produced barley and loved the corn-god; the Nile greeted me on every . . .[2] None hungered in my years, none thirsted in them. Men dwelt (in peace) through that which I wrought and talked of me (?); all that I commanded was as it should be.

I tamed (?) lions and captured crocodiles.[3] I . . . ed the Wawa,[4] and captured the Matoï;[4] I caused the Bedouins to go as dogs.[5] I built an house adorned with gold; its ceilings are of lapis lazuli [6] . . ., its floor is . . ., the doors are of copper and the bolts of bronze, they are made for endless time, and eternity is afraid of them.[7]

The schoolboy, on whose scribblings we are at this juncture almost entirely dependent, has so utterly garbled the conclusion, that we can only make out disconnected scraps: There is much talk in the streets. I know: " Yea " and make search because of its beauty, for he knoweth it not [8] – – – – King Sesōstris. Thy feet go. Thou art mine own heart, mine eyes gaze upon (thee). The children have an hour of happiness beside the people, when they give thee praise.

Behold, I have wrought at the beginning, and thou (?) commandest at the end – – – – the white crown of the divine seed.[9]

There is exultation in the boat of Rē.– – – –[10] Monuments are set up and thy tomb (?) is made splendid – – – –.

---

[1] The southern frontier town.
[2] The inundation reached even the most inaccessible places.
[3] Probably figurative for foreign peoples.
[4] Nubian people.
[5] So docile were they.
[6] *I.e.* the ceilings of the rooms are painted to represent the sky.
[7] Because it sees that it will never be able to destroy them.
[8] The whole of this meaningless sentence, as can be seen only, it is true, in the original, is derived from the verse of the *Admonitions* (p. 100), " Nay, but the children of the magistrates are thrown on to the streets. He that hath knowledge saith: ' Yea.' The fool saith: ' Nay.' He that hath no knowledge, to him seemeth it good."
[9] The king.
[10] See GUNN, *Syntax*, p. 148.

The Ancient Egyptian Wisdom Texts
The Teachings of Sage Ani

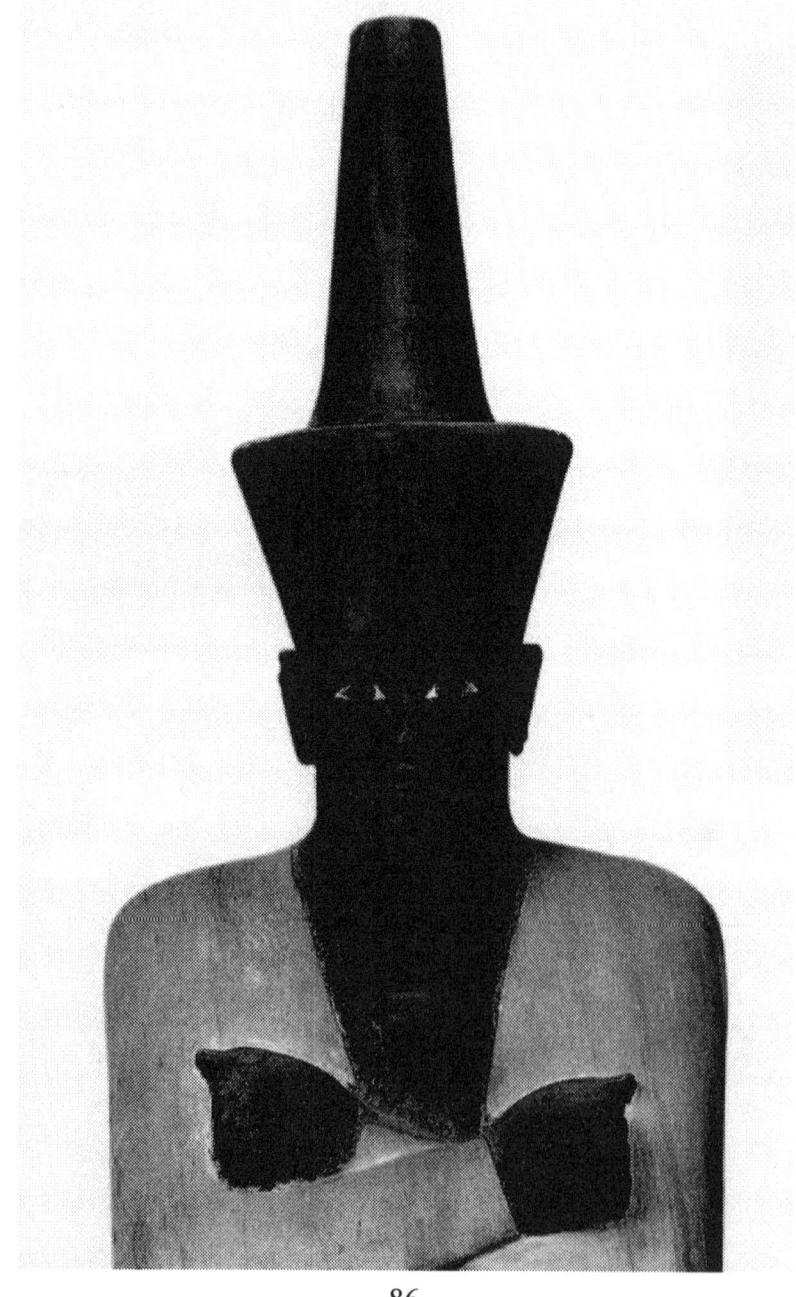

The Ancient Egyptian Wisdom Texts

THE WISDOM OF ANII [7]

This book is a late imitation of the old books of wisdom, and resembles them in this respect also, that in it, as in them, a father is propounding his teaching to his son. But the scope of this work seems to be wider and its tone livelier—I say "seems," for, unfortunately, unless a new manuscript turns up, we shall never be able to understand more than isolated fragments of this wisdom. The schoolboy, who copied out the papyrus, has made mistakes in the writing of most of the words, and for the length of whole passages one has absolutely no idea of what is the subject under discussion. Possibly he did not understand much of what his book contained, for although it is written in New Egyptian, this language already belonged to a period separated some three to four hundred years from a schoolboy of the Twenty-First or Twenty-Second Dynasty, and thus much of it might have been obscure to him. We have evidence, moreover, that this was actually the case. The Berlin Museum possesses the writing-equipment of a schoolboy, who likewise lived in the Twenty-Second Dynasty, comprising a writing-board,[8] upon which are written what were originally the opening words of our book. And yet he already had to add to these words a rendering in the language that was familiar to him. "Beginning of the exhortatory instruction (the commencement of the exhortatory instructions) composed by the scribe Anii (which the scribe Anii composed) of the house of Nefer(ke)rē-teri." With this last name we might possibly associate a similarly named king at the end of the Old Kingdom, and suppose that the author of the work wished to place his sage in that period, although he gave him and his son names belonging to the New Kingdom.

---

[1] Who speak entirely different dialects. Meaning: your style is so unintelligible.

[2] Of the Palace.

[3] Meaning, probably: In your high position you need not write clearly, for it is all good in the eyes of those who read it.

[4] Palestine. [5] Be friendly.

[6] Be not wroth, but be glad to learn from me.

[7] Papyrus of the Twenty-Second Dynasty in Cairo; published by Chabas in 1874 in the periodical, *L'Égyptologie*, under the title of *Les maximes du scribe Ani*.

[8] *Zeitschr. für ägypt. Sprache*, xxxii. p. 127.

The Ancient Egyptian Wisdom Texts

[FOLLOW MY WORDS.]
(I tell thee) that which is excellent, that which thou shalt observe (?) in thine heart. Do it, *and so thou wilt be good*, and all evil is far from thee. – – – – *It will be said of thee :* a good character, *and not* : he is ruined, he is idle. *Accept my words*, and so will all evil be far from thee.

[BE PRUDENT IN SPEECH ?]
Unintelligible.

[BE RETICENT.]
Guard thyself against ought that injureth (?) great people, by talking of secret affairs. If (anyone) speaketh (of them) in thine house, make (thyself ?) deaf – – – –.

[BOAST NOT OF THY STRENGTH ?]
Unintelligible.

[FOUND A FAMILY.]
Take to thyself a wife when thou art a youth, that she may give thee a son. Thou shouldest beget him for thee whilst thou art yet young, *and shouldest live to see* him become a man (?). Happy is the man who hath much people, and he is respected because of his children (?).

[BE PIOUS.]
Celebrate the feast of thy god – – – –. God is wroth with him that disregardeth it. Let witnesses stand by thine offering; it is best (?) for him that hath done it (?) – – – – Singing, dancing, and frankincense appertain to his maintenance (?), and the receiving of reverence appertaineth to his possessions.[1] Bestow them on the god in order to magnify his name – – – –.

[1] God has a right to be reverenced.

The Ancient Egyptian Wisdom Texts

[BE DISCREET ON VISITS.]

Enter not the (house ?) of another, – – – –. Gaze not on that which is not right in (his ?) house ; thine eye may see it, but thou keepest silent. Speak not of it to another outside, that it may not become for thee a great crime worthy of death, when it is heard (?).

[BEWARE OF THE HARLOT.]

Beware of a strange woman, one that is not known in her city. Wink (?) not at her – – – – have no carnal knowledge of her (?). (She is) a deep water whose twisting men know not.[1] A woman that is far from her husband, " I am fair," she saith to thee every day, when she hath no witnesses – – – –. It is a great crime worthy of death, when one heareth of it, and although it is not related outside – – – –.

[BE RESERVED IN THY CONDUCT.]

Go not in and out in the court of justice, that thy name may not stink – – – –. Speak not much, be silent, that thou mayest be happy. Be not a gossip.

[THE TRUE PIETY.]

The dwelling of God, it abhorreth clamour. Pray with a loving heart, all the words whereof are hidden. Then he will do what thou needest ; he will hear what thou sayest and accept thine offering.

[PIETY TOWARDS PARENTS.]

Offer water to thy father and thy mother, who rest in the desert-valley – – – –. Omit not to do it, that thy son may do the like for thee.

[BE NOT A DRUNKARD.]

Take not upon thyself (?)[2] to drink a jug of beer. Thou speakest, and an unintelligible utterance issueth from thy mouth. If thou fallest down and thy limbs break, there is none to hold out a hand to thee. Thy companions in drink stand up and say : " *Away with this sot !* " If there (then) cometh one to

[1] The changing current ? eddy ?
[2] Possible meaning : Boast not that you can drink, etc.

seek thee in order to question thee, thou art found lying on the ground, and thou art like a little child.

[Lead an honest life?]
Go not forth from thine house to one that thou knowest not (?) – – – – let every place that thou favourest be known.

[Be mindful of death.]
Make for thyself a fair abode in the desert-valley, the deep which will hide thy corpse. Have it before thine eyes in thine occupations – – – – even as (?) the great elders, who rest in their sepulchre (?). He who maketh it (for himself) meeteth with no reproof; good is it if thou too art furnished in like manner. Thy messenger[1] cometh to thee – – – – *he placeth himself in front of thee (?)*. Say not: "I am too young for thee to carry off," for thou knowest not thy death. Death cometh and leadeth away the babe that is still in the bosom of its mother, even as the man when he hath become old.

Here begins a fresh section of some length, in which, firstly, caution in social intercourse is enjoined—most of it frankly unintelligible.

Behold, I tell thee yet other excellent things, which thou shalt heed (?) in thine heart. Do them, and thou wilt be happy, and all evil will be far from thee – – – –.

[Caution in social intercourse.]
Keep thyself far from an hostile man, and take him not to thee for a companion. Make to thyself a friend (rather) of one that is upright and righteous, when thou seest what he hath done (?) – – – –.

Make not a friend of the slave of another, whose name stinketh – – – –. If one pursueth him in order to seize him, and to take away him that is in his house, thou art wretched and sayest: "What am I to do?" – – – –

[Possessions do not make for happiness?]
A man constructeth a house for himself. A piece of ground (?) is laid out for thee, thou hast fenced in (?) a garden of herbs in front of thine arable land; thou hast planted sycamores inside – – – – and thou fillest thine hand with all

[1] Probably meaning Death, who comes to summon you.

The Ancient Egyptian Wisdom Texts

flowers that thine eye perceiveth. (But) with them all one is wretched – – – –.

Put not thy trust in the possessions of another; guard thyself *from doing that* (?). Rely not on the things of another – – – – say not: "The father of my mother hath an house – – – –. For *when it cometh to the* division with thy brethren, thy share (is only) a storehouse. If thy god grants that a child be born to thee – – – –.

[BE RESPECTFUL.]
Sit not when another standeth, one that is older than thou, or that hath occupied himself in his calling longer than thou – – – –.

The subject with which the passages immediately following are concerned, cannot even be conjectured.

[USEFULNESS OF KNOWLEDGE.]
Men do all that thou sayest, if thou art skilled in the writings. Devote thyself to the writings, and put them in thine heart, and then all that thou sayest is excellent. To whatsoever office the scribe is appointed, he consulteth the writings.[1] There is no son for the superintendent of the treasury, no heir for the superintendent of the fortress – – – – the offices, which have no children – – – –.[2]

[BE CAUTIOUS IN SPEECH.]
Speak not out thine heart to the . . . man – – – –. A wrong word that hath come forth from thy mouth, if (he?) repeateth it, thou makest enemies (for thyself). A man falleth in ruin because of his tongue – – – –. A man's belly is broader than a granary, and is full of all manner of answers. Choose thou out the good and speak them, while the bad remain imprisoned in thy belly. – – – –

Of a truth thou will ever be with me and answer him that injureth me with falsehood, in spite of God who judgeth the righteous. His fate cometh to carry him off.[3]

[1] Through them he is always successful and is therefore fit to succeed to any office, as is amplified in what follows.
[2] The most worthy obtains them, *i.e.* he who has learnt most.
[3] If the sentence is to be thus translated, the sage is here referring to some wrong which had been done him by an enemy, and of which an account may have been given in the lost beginning of the book.

The Ancient Egyptian Wisdom Texts

[Relations with God.]

Make offering to thy god and keep thyself from trespassing against him. Inquire not concerning his form ; *walk not with swaggering gait,* when he goeth forth in procession ; press not forward to carry him.[1] – – – – Let thine eye mark how he is wroth, *and have respect for* his name. It is he that giveth power (?) to millions of forms, and (only) he is made great whom he maketh great. The god of this land is the sun which is in the horizon, (but) his images are on earth ; *to them let incense be offered daily.*

[Be grateful to thy mother.]

Double the bread that thou givest to thy mother, and carry her as she carried (thee). She had a heavy load in thee, and never left it to me.[2] When thou wast born after thy months, she carried thee yet again about her neck, and for three years her breast was in thy mouth. *She was not* disgusted at thy dung, she was not disgusted and said not : " What do I ? " She put thee to school, when thou hadst been taught to write, and daily she stood there . . .[3] with bread and beer from her house.

When thou art a young man and takest to thee a wife and art settled in thine house, keep before thee how thy mother gave birth to thee, and how she brought thee up further in all manner of ways. May she not do thee harm nor lift up her hands to God, and may he not hear her cry.

[On wealth and its instability.]

Eat not bread, if another is suffering want, and thou dost not stretch out the hand to him with bread. – – – –. One is rich and another is poor – – – –. He that was rich in past years, is this year a groom. Be not greedy about filling thy belly – – – –. The course of the water of last year, it is this year in another place. Great seas have become dry places, and banks have become abysses. – – – –

[On paying visits ?]

Go not freely to a man in (his) house, but enter in (only) when thou art bidden. When he hath said to thee " Praise to

---

[1] In the procession.
[2] I (thy father) could not help her.   [3] *I.e.* outside the school.

The Ancient Egyptian Wisdom Texts

thee" with his mouth, – – – –. *Then after an unintelligible passage:* give him to God and give him daily again to God. The morrow is as to-day. Thou wilt see what God will do, if he besmircheth (?) him that hath besmirched (?) thee.[1]

[KEEP THYSELF FAR FROM TUMULTS.]

Enter not into a crowd, if thou findest *that it standeth ready for* beating – – – – that thou mayest not be blamed in the Court before the magistrates after the tendering of evidence, Keep thee far from hostile people – – – –.

[TREAT THY WIFE WELL.]

Act not the official over thy wife in her house, if thou knowest that she is excellent. Say not unto her: "Where is it? Bring it us," if (?) she hath put (it) in the right place. Let thine eye observe and be silent, that so (?) thou mayest know her good deeds. (She is) happy when thine hand is with her – – – –. Thereby the man ceaseth to stir up strife in his house – – – –.

[BE CAREFUL OF WOMEN.]

Go not after a woman, in order that she may not steal thine heart away.[2]

[BEHAVIOUR TOWARDS SUPERIORS.]

Answer not a superior who is enraged, *get out of his way.* Say what is sweet, when he saith what is bitter to any one, and make calm his heart. Contentious answers carry rods,[3] and thy strength collapseth. *Rage directeth itself* (?) against thy business, *therefore vex (?) not thine own self.* He turneth about and praiseth thee quickly, after his terrible hour. If thy words are soothing for the heart, the heart inclineth to receive them. Seek out silence for thyself, and submit to what he doeth.

[STAND WELL WITH THE POLICE.]

Make a friend of the herald[4] of thy quarter, and let him not become enraged with thee. Give him dainties when there

---

[1] Might apply to some one who had committed a wrong, the punishment of whom let God see to?

[2] Probably only the beginning of a section.

[3] Lead to thy being beaten.

[4] Here and elsewhere merely the title of an official.

The Ancient Egyptian Wisdom Texts

are any in thine house,[1] and pass him not by at his prayers. Say to him: " Praise to thee " – – – –.

An unintelligible passage is followed by a dialogue, with which the book concludes.

The scribe Khenshotep answered his father, the scribe Anii: " Ah, would that I were *as thou (?)* – – – – so would (?) I act in accordance with thy teaching, that (?) the son should be promoted to his father's place – – – –. *Thou art a man* with lofty desires, all of whose words are choice. *A son that* imagineth (?) *evil within himself,* he saith – – – – in books. Thy words are soothing for mine heart, and mine heart inclineth to receive them. Mine heart rejoiceth. (But) let not thine excellence be too abundant, – – – – a boy *doth not yet do* according to the teaching that instructs, albeit (?) the books are on his tongue."[2]

The scribe Anii answered his son, the scribe Khenshotep: " Trust not in these hazardous things (?). *Avoid further complaining, mine heart heedeth it not.* Even the fighting bull, that hath slain the stall,[3] cannot leave the ring, *and receiveth* his instructions *from the* drover. The fierce lion abateth his rage and doefully passeth by the ass. The horse submitteth to his yoke – – – – –. The dog, he hearkeneth to words and followeth his master. The kaeri-animal[4] carrieth the . . . vessel, which his mother carried not. The goose alighteth on the cool pool, when it is chased, and then fretteth itself in the net. Negroes are taught to speak Egyptian, and Syrians, and all strangers likewise. *I too have discoursed on* all the callings that thou mayest hear, and know what is to be done."

What the son replies to this is unintelligible; he probably alludes to the fact that most men are worthless. There is a multitude of all that is evil (?), and none knoweth his teaching. If there be one that is prudent, the bulk is *foolish. He then probably would vow obedience to his father:* All thy words are excellent – – – – I give thee oaths, place them upon thy way.

The scribe Anii answered his son, the scribe Khenshotep: " Turn thy back on these many words, which are far from being heard. The bent (?) stick that lieth in the field, *exposed*

[1] On festival days.
[2] The meaning of the whole passage may be: Go not too far in thy demands, or else, though I may carry thy wisdom in my mouth, I shall not conduct myself in accordance with it.
[3] The other oxen of the stall.   [4] See above, p. 189, note 5.

The Ancient Egyptian Wisdom Texts

to (?) sun and shade, the craftsman fetcheth it and maketh it straight, and maketh it into the whip of a notable. But the straight piece of wood, that maketh he into a board (?).[1] O heart that cannot deliberate, is it thy will to give oaths, or dost thou miscarry ? "

Anii then probably expresses the hope that his son, who already knoweth the strength in his hand,[2] *may be as sensible as* the child in its mother's arms. *When it cometh to years of discretion and no longer wishes to suck,* it findeth its mouth in order to say: " Give me bread."

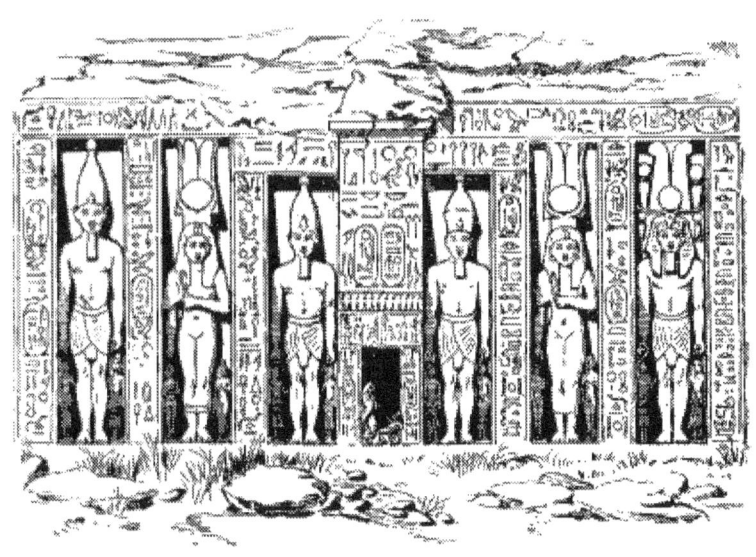

[1] Meaning probably: one can train every one, but the result is of varying value. It remains doubtful, however, whether the sage gives the preference to the beautiful whip or the level board.

[2] *I.e.* feels himself strong.

The Ancient Egyptian Wisdom Texts

The Teachings of Duauf

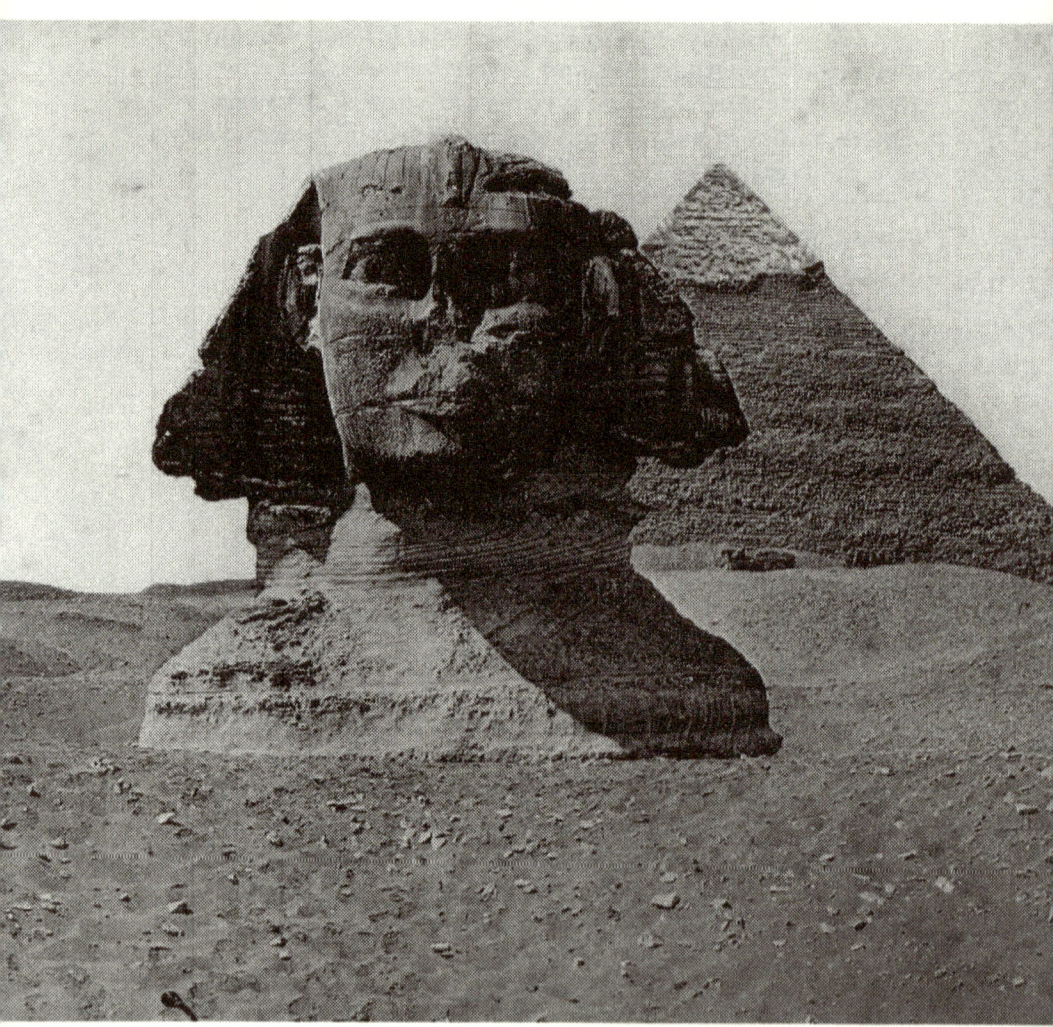

The Ancient Egyptian Wisdom Texts

This *Instruction* was a favourite work in the schools of the late New Kingdom, and it is, moreover, preserved only in schoolboys' exercises of the Nineteenth Dynasty (about 1300 B.C.) — completely in two papyri, and in parts on several ostraca. The way in which the boys have mangled the text baffles description. There are not many passages in it with regard to which one does not despairingly ask what can have been written there originally ; for what the boys have written are only too often meaningless words—they simply did not understand what they had to copy out. Of many paragraphs, therefore, I can only translate a small portion.

It is not surprising that this work was such a favourite school textbook, for it is written to extol schools and a school-education, exactly as are the fictitious letters to and from schoolmasters in the New Kingdom. It can be seen from the personal names con-

---

[1] They regulated their behaviour in accordance with it.
[2] Usual euphemism for " to die."
[3] Preserved in *Pap. Sallier*, ii. and *Pap. Anastasi*, vii. in the British Museum. Brought to light by Goodwin in 1858 ; edited by MASPERO, *Genre épistolaire*, pp. 48 ff. A recent edition is wanting.

The Ancient Egyptian Wisdom Texts

tained in this *Instruction*, that it is to be dated to the time between the Old and Middle Kingdoms.

Instruction, which a . . . man,[1] named Duauf, the son of Khety, composed for his son, named Pepi, when he voyaged up to the Residence, in order to put him in the School of Books, *among* the children of the magistrates – – – –.

He said unto him: I have seen him that is beaten, him that is beaten: thou art to set thine heart on books. I have beheld him that is set free from forced labour: behold, nothing surpasseth books.[2]

Read at the end of the Kemit;[3] thou findest this sentence therein: "The scribe, his is every place at the Residence and he is not poor in it.[4] *But he that acteth according to* the understanding of another,[5] *he hath no success.*" *The other professions also are* as this sentence purporteth.

Would that I might make thee love books more than thy mother, would that I might bring their beauty before thy face. It is greater than any calling. – – – – If he[6] hath begun to succeed, and is yet a child, men greet him.[7] He is sent to carry out behests, and he cometh not home that he may don the apron.[8]

Never have I seen a sculptor on an errand, nor a goldsmith as he was being sent forth. But I have seen the smith at his task at the mouth of his furnace. His fingers were like stuff from crocodiles,[9] he stank more than the offal (?) of fishes.

Every artisan that wieldeth the chisel (?), he is wearier than he that delveth; his field is the wood and his hoe is the metal.[10] In the night, when he is set free, he worketh beyond what his arms can do; in the night he burneth a light.[11]

The stone-mason seeketh for work (?) in all manner of hard stone. *When he hath finished it*, his arms *are* destroyed and

---

[1] Apparently a person of low standing.

[2] The uneducated is faced with a life of flogging, the educated need not do any rough work.

[3] Is this the name of some old book?

[4] Meaning probably: Every office which a scribe fills is in connection with the court, and so the scribe has a share before others in all the favours which are distributed there.

[5] Thus is himself not a learned official.   [6] The schoolboy.

[7] So soon do men begin to treat him with deference.

[8] The "apron" here and further on will denote the clothing of the artisan.

[9] As crinkled and hard as their skin.   [10] *I.e.* the chisel.

[11] Even at night there is no respite for him.

The Ancient Egyptian Wisdom Texts

he is weary. When such an one sitteth down at dusk, his thighs and his back are broken.

The barber shaveth late into the evening – – – –, he betaketh him from street to street, in order to seek (?) whom he may shave. *He straineth his arms* in order to fill his belly, even as a bee that feedeth at its work.[1]

The . . . sails down to the Delta in order to get the purchase-money,[2] and he worketh beyond that his arms can do. The gnats[3] slay him – – – –.

The small bricklayer[4] with the Nile mud (?), he spendeth his life among the cattle (?) ; *he is somehow concerned with* vines *and* swine,[5] his clothes are stiff, – – – – *he worketh* (?) with his feet, he poundeth – – – –.

Let me tell thee further of the builder of walls, *that is ofttimes sick (?), his raiment is likewise vile; what he eateth is* the bread of his fingers *and* he washeth himself once only. — *He fares so ill that the sage has to devote a second paragraph to him, of which only a little is intelligible to us :*

He is more miserable than one can rightly tell (?). *He is like a block of stone (?)* in a room, which measureth ten cubits by six cubits. – – – – The bread, he giveth it unto his house ; his children are beaten, beaten.

The gardener bringeth loads,[6] *and his arm and neck ache beneath them.* At morn he watereth the leek, and at even the vines – – – –. *It also goeth more ill with him than* any calling.

The field-worker, his reckoning endureth for ever ;[7] he hath a louder voice than the abu-bird – – – –. *He, too,* is wearier than can be told (?), *and* he fareth as well as one fareth among lions ; *he is oft-times sick (?),* – – – – *and* when he cometh unto his house at eventide, the going hath cut him to pieces (?).[8]

---

[1] As indefatigably as it collects honey.   [2] Thus a trader ?
[3] The pest of the Delta.
[4] This seems to be the bricklayer who makes brick out of Nile mud and builds with them.
[5] In the Egyptian there is a play on the words " vines " and " swine," and it is probably on that account that they are brought together here.
[6] The produce of the garden.
[7] Probably the settling up of accounts with the owner, so often depicted in the old tombs ; the standing jokes in the scenes being that the peasants talk a great deal and get a hiding.
[8] The long roads have worn him out ?

The Ancient Egyptian Wisdom Texts

The weaver (?) in the workshop, he fareth more ill than any women.[1] His thighs are upon his belly,[2] and he breatheth no air. *On a day, when no weaving is done, he must* pluck (?) lotus flowers in the pond. He giveth bread to the doorkeeper,[3] that he may suffer him to come into the daylight.

The fletcher, he fareth ill exceedingly, when he goeth up into the desert.[4] Much giveth he for his ass, much giveth he for what is in the field.[5] When he setteth out on the road (?) – – – – and cometh unto his house at eventime, the going hath cut him to pieces (?).

The . . . goeth up into the desert, and (first) maketh over his goods to his children, for fear of the lions and the Asiatics – – – – and cometh unto his house at eventide, the going hath cut him to pieces (?) – – – –.

The . . ., his fingers stink, and the odour thereof is abhorrent (?) – – – –. He spendeth the day cutting reed, and clothes are his abhorrence.[6]

The cobbler, he fareth ill exceedingly; he beggeth ever. He fareth as well as one fareth among . . . What he biteth is leather.[7]

The fuller washeth upon the river bank, a near neighbour of the crocodile – – – –. This is no peaceful calling in thine eyes, that would be more tranquil than all callings – – – –.

The fowler, he fareth ill exceedingly, when he looketh at the birds in the sky. When the passers-by [8] are joined to the heaven, he saith: " Would that I had a net here." *But God giveth him no success (?)*.

Let me tell thee further, how it fareth with the fisherman; it goeth more ill with him than any other calling. Is not his work upon the river, where he is mixed with the crocodiles? – – – –. One saith not: " There is a crocodile there "; fear

---

[1] Who also must always sit in the house.
[2] He squats on the ground on his haunches.   [3] He bribes him.
[4] Where he fashions the arrow-heads out of the quantities of flints that are to be found there.
[5] The donkey's fodder.   [6] Because he is standing in the water.
[7] He uses his teeth at his work in order to pull tight the sandal-straps, as he is actually shown doing in a scene on a tomb wall (ROSELLINI, *Mon. Civili.*, lxiv. 1). The jest obviously is that this is the only thing that comes between his teeth.
[8] The migratory birds, which formed a substantial item in the food-supply of the Egyptians.

The Ancient Egyptian Wisdom Texts

hath blinded him – – – –. Behold, there is no calling that is without a director except (that of) the scribe, and he is the director.[1]

If he knoweth the books, then true of him is : " They are good for thee " – – – –. *What I now do* on the voyage up to the Residence, lo, I do it out of love for thee. A day at school is profitable to thee, *and its work endureth even like the mountains* – – – –.

Most of what is to be found in the following sections is unintelligible. As the introduction to them shows : Let me say to thee further yet other words in order to instruct thee, *they deal with a new theme ; indeed, they may be a later addition.* The one section teaches good behaviour in the presence of the great : If thou enterest, while the master of the house is in his house, *and he hath to do with another first,* while thou sittest with thine hand to thy mouth, ask not for anything. *Further :* Speak no hidden words *and* speak no insolent words – – – –. *Then :* If thou comest from school and midday is announced to thee, and thou goest shouting joyously in the streets, then – – – –. If a great man sendeth thee with a message,[2] *repeat it as he saith it ;* take nothing therefrom and add nothing thereto – – – –.

Be content with thy diet : If three loaves satisfy thee, and thou drinkest two pots of beer, *and the belly is not yet contented, fight against it* (?).

Behold, it is good if thou sendest away the multitude and hearkenest (alone) to the words of the great. – – – – Make a friend of a man of thy generation.

Behold, Renenet [3] is upon the way of God ; Renenet, the scribe hath her upon his arm on the day of his birth.[4] He

head of the officials is he set, and his father and his mother thank God *for it* – – – –. Behold, this it is *that I set before thee and thy children's children.*

[1] This thought is the culmination of all that the sage has hitherto been saying.
[2] In the school or on the way home ?
[3] The goddess of the harvest ; the following sentences assert somehow or other that *a scribe never suffers want.*
[4] This will have some connection with the custom, which we know from statues, of having the name of one's master either branded or tattoed on the upper part of the arm. So the scribe is the property of the goddess, who gives plentiful sustenance.
[5] The goddess of birth, see p. 44, note 2.

The Ancient Egyptian Wisdom Texts

The Teachings of Merikara

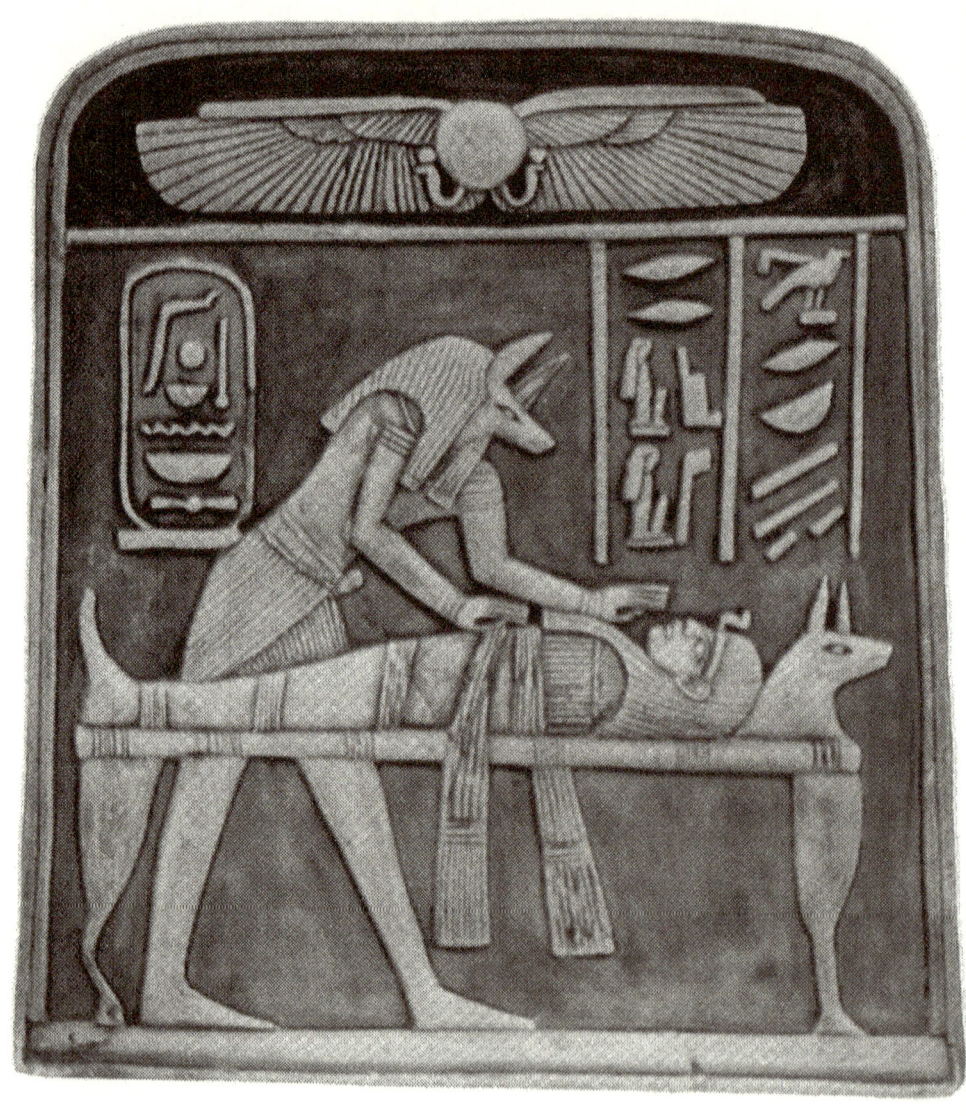

The Ancient Egyptian Wisdom Texts

The Instructions To Merikara

Introduction

The following is a rendition of an Ancient Egyptian Wisdom text commonly known as *The Instructions To Merikara*. It is written in the form of instructions being passed down from a ruling king to an heir, a teacher to the disciple. They contain profound teachings referring to the nature of the Divine, Creation, human psychology and spiritual evolution in life. Therefore, with careful study and reflection, the verses of this text reveal important mystical wisdom which when understood and practiced will lead to peace and prosperity in the world of human existence as well as inner spiritual peace and contentment. The line numbers have been added for the purpose of referencing and commentary.

The Instructions To Merikara are written in the form of a teaching given from a reigning king to the prince or heir apparent. The underlying theme is one of a Teacher-Disciple relationship. Anyone who rises to a position of management or as a teacher in society is as royalty. Moving out of a stage of life which is of the masses puts one in a minority of those who manage and lead society. Therefore, the teachings have a practical level for those who would like to provide guidance in society and to promote peace and well being therein.

There is another important element in The Instructions To Merikara. This involves the psychology of human nature. It is a teaching that places importance in understanding the difference between virtuous character and vicious character. The vicious development in humanity is the source of strife in society. The virtuous development is the source of harmony and spiritual enlightenment.

The Ancient Egyptian Wisdom Texts

THE INSTRUCTIONS TO MERIKARA

(1) The hothead incites citizens; He creates divisions among the young; If you see that people follow him,

(2) Speak out against him before those who give council, Suppress the hothead, he is against harmony, The talker is a troublemaker for society. Your duty is to curb the multitude, and suppress its heat...

(3) May you be justified before The God,
That a man may say of you even when you are absent,
That you punish in accordance [with what is just for the crime].
Good nature allows a man to experience heaven,
The cursing of the [angry and agitated ones] is painful to oneself.

(4) If you are skilled in the art of speech, you will prevail, The tongue is [a leader or wise person's] sword;
Speaking rightly is more powerful than all fighting, The skillful in speech (ethics-philosophy) cannot be overcome.

(5) The wise one is a [teacher] to the nobles.
Those who know that he knows will not attack him, No [crime or injustice] occurs when a wise one is near; justice comes to them distilled,
In the form of the sayings of the ancestors.
Copy your fathers, your ancestors,

(6) See that the their wise words endure in books,
Open them and read them, copy their knowledge, they who are taught become skilled.
Don't act with evil, kindness is an expression of good nature,
Make your memory last through love of you.
Increase the [people], befriend the town,
God will be praised for (your) donations,
One will ------
Praise your goodness,
Pray for your health

The Ancient Egyptian Wisdom Texts

(7) Respect the nobles, sustain your people,

(8) Strengthen your borders, your frontier patrols; It is good to work for the future,
One respects the life of the foresighted,
While he who trusts fails.
Make people come [to you] through your good nature, A wretch is who desires the land [of his neighbor],
A fool is who covets what others possess.
(9) A million men do not benefit the Lord of the Two Lands. Is there [a man] who lives forever?
He who comes with Osiris passes,
He leaves those who indulged themselves.
Advance your officials, so that they act by your laws,
The one who has wealth at home will not be partial,
He is a just man who lacks nothing.
The poor man does not speak justly,
Not righteous is one who says, "I wish I had,"

(10) Great is the great man whose great men are great,
Strong is the king who has righteous councilors,
Wealthy is he who is rich in his nobles acquaintances.

(11) Speak truth in your house,
That the officials of the land may respect you; Uprightness befits the lord,
The front of the house puts fear in the back.

(12) Do justice, then you endure on earth;
Calm the weeper, don't oppress the widow, Don't expel a man from his father's property; Don't reduce the nobles in their possessions. Beware of punishing wrongfully,
Do not kill, it does not serve you.
Punish with beatings, with detention,
Thus will the land be well ordered;
Except for the unrighteous one whose plans are found out,

(13) For god knows the treason plotters,
God smites the rebels in blood. He who is merciful --- lifetime;

The Ancient Egyptian Wisdom Texts

Do not kill a man whose virtues you know,
With whom you once chanted the writings,
Who was brought up.... before God,
Who strode freely in the secret place.*
The *ba* comes to the place it knows,
It does not miss its former path,
No kind of magic holds it back,
It comes to those who give it water.*

(14) The Court that judges the wretch,
You know they are not lenient,
On the day of judging the miserable,
In the hour of doing their task.
It is painful when the accuser has knowledge,
Do not trust in length of years,
They view a lifetime in an hour!
When a man remains over after death,
His deeds are set beside him as treasure,
And being yonder lasts forever.
A fool is who does what they reprove!
He who reaches them without having done wrong
 Will exist there like a god,
Free-striding like the lords forever!

(15) Raise your youths and the residence will love you,
Increase your subjects with friendship,
See, your city is full of new growth.
Twenty years the youths indulge their wishes, Then they go forth as [recruits]...
Veterans return to their children ...

I raised troops from them on my accession. Advance your officials, promote your [soldiers],
Enrich the young men who follow you,
Provide them with goods, endow them with fields,
Reward them with herds.

The Ancient Egyptian Wisdom Texts

(16) Do not prefer the well born to the commoner,
Choose a man on account of his skills,
Then all crafts are done --- . . .
Guard your borders, secure your forts,
Troops are useful to their lord.

(17) Make your monuments [worthy] of The God, This keeps alive their maker's name,
A man should do what profits his *ba*.
In the monthly service, wear the white sandals, Visit the temple, discover the mysteries,
Enter the shrine, eat bread in God's house; Proffer libations, multiply the loaves,
Make ample the daily offerings,
It profits him who does it.
Endow your monuments according to your wealth,
Even one day of spiritual practice leads to eternity,
Even an hour contributes to the future,
God recognizes the one who works for Him.

(18) Troops will fight troops
As the ancestors foretold;
Egypt fought in the graveyard,
Destroying tombs in vengeful destruction.
As I did it, so it happened,
As is done to one who strays from god's path. Do not deal evilly with the Southland,
You know what the residence foretold about it; As this happened so that may happen.
Before they had trespassed- - -
I attacked This [straight to] its southern border at [Taut]-,
I engulfed it like a flood;
King Meriyebre, justified, had not done it;
Be merciful on account of it,
------ renew the treaties.

(19) No river lets itself be hidden,
It is good to work for the future.

The Ancient Egyptian Wisdom Texts

You stand well with the Southland,
They come to you with tribute, with gifts;
I have acted like the forefathers:
If one has no grain to give,
Be kind, since they are humble before you.
Be sated with your bread, your beer,
Granite comes to you unhindered.
Do not despoil the monument of another,

(20) But quarry stone in Tura.
Do not build your tomb out of ruins,
(Using) what had been made for what is to be made.
Behold, the king is lord of joy,

(21) You may rest, sleep in your strength,
Follow your heart, through what I have done,
There is no foe within your borders.
I   arose as lord of the city,
Whose heart was sad because of the Northland;
From Hetshenu to [Sembaqa], and south to Two-Fish Channel.
I pacified the entire West as far as the coast of the sea.
It pays taxes, it gives cedar wood,"
One sees juniper wood which they give us.
The East abounds in bowmen,
The inner islands are turned back,
And every man within,

(22) The temples say, "you are greater than I."
The land they had ravaged has been made into nomes,
All kinds of large towns [are in it-];
What was ruled by one is in the hands of ten, Officials are appointed, tax [lists drawn up].

(23) When free men are given land,
They work for you like a single team;
No rebel will arise among them,
And Hapi will not fail to come.
The dues of the Northland are in your hand,

The Ancient Egyptian Wisdom Texts

For the mooring-post is staked in the district I made in the East
From Hebenu to Horusway;
It is settled with towns, filled with people,
Of the best in the whole land,
To repel attacks against them.
May I see a brave man who will copy it,
Who will add to what I have done,
A wretched heir would disgrace me.

(24) But this should be said to the Bowman:
Lo, the miserable Asiatic,
He is wretched because of the place he's in:
Short of water, bare of wood,
Its paths are many and painful because of mountains.
He does not dwell in one place,
Food propels his legs,
He fights since the time of Horus,
Not conquering nor being conquered,
He does not announce the day of combat,
Like a thief who darts about a group.
But as I live and shall be what I am,
When the Bowmen were a sealed wall,
I breached [their strongholds],
I made Lower Egypt attack them,
I captured their inhabitants,
I seized their cattle,
Until the Asiatics abhorred Egypt.
Do not concern yourself with him,
The Asiatic is a crocodile on its shore,
It snatches from a lonely road,
It cannot seize from a populous town.

(25) Medenyt has been restored to its Nome,
Its one side is irrigated as far as Kem-Wer,
It is the defense [against] the Bowmen.
Its walls are warlike, its soldiers many,
Its serfs know how to bear arms,
Apart from the free men within.

The Ancient Egyptian Wisdom Texts

The region of Memphis totals ten thousand men,
Free citizens who are not taxed;
Officials are in it since the time it was residence,
The borders are firm, the garrisons valiant.
Many northerners irrigate it as far as the Northland,
Taxed with grain in the manner of free men;
Lo, it is the gateway of the Northland,
They form a dike as far as Hnes.
Abundant citizens are the heart's support,

(26) Beware of being surrounded by the serfs of the foe,
Caution prolongs life.
If your southern border is attacked,
The Bowmen will put on the girdle,

(27) Build buildings in the Northland!
As a man's name is not made small by his actions,
So a settled town is not harmed.
Build ------
The foe loves destruction and misery.
King Khety, the justified, laid down in teaching:
He who is <u>silent</u> toward violence diminishes the offerings.
God will attack the rebel for the sake of the temple,
He will be overcome for what he has done,
He will be sated with what he planned to gain,
He will find no favor on the day of woe.
Supply the offerings, revere The God,
Don't say, "it is trouble," don't slacken your hands.
He who opposes you attacks the sky,
A monument is sound for a hundred years;
If the foe understood, he would not attack them,
There is no one who has no enemy.

(28) The Lord of the Two Shores is one who knows,
A king who has courtiers is not ignorant;
As one wise did he come from the womb,
From a million men God singled him out.

The Ancient Egyptian Wisdom Texts

A goodly office is kingship,
It has no son, no brother to maintain its memorial,
But one man provides for the other;
A man acts for him who was before him,
So that what he has done is preserved by his successor.
Lo, a shameful deed occurred in my time:
The Nome of This was ravaged;
Though it happened during my reign,
I learned it after it was done.
There was retribution for what was done,
For it is evil to destroy,
Useless to restore what one has damaged,
To rebuild what one has demolished.
Beware of it! A blow is repaid by its like,
To every action there is a response.

(29) While generation succeeds generation,
God who knows characters is hidden;
One can not oppose the lord of the hand,
He reaches all that the eyes can see.

(30) One should revere The God on his path,
Made of costly stone, fashioned of bronze.
As watercourse is replaced by watercourse,
So no river allows itself to be concealed,
It breaks the channel in which it was hidden.
So also the *ba* goes to the place it knows,
And strays not from its former path.
Make firm your station in the graveyards,
By being upright, by doing justice,
Upon which men's hearts rely.
The loaf of the upright is preferred
To the ox of the evildoer.
Work for God, He will work for you also,
With offerings that make the altar flourish,
With carvings that proclaim your name,
God thinks of him who works for him.

The Ancient Egyptian Wisdom Texts

(31) Well tended is humankind-god's cattle,
He made sky and earth for their sake,
He subdued the water monster,
He made breath for their noses to live.
They are His images, who came from His body,
He shines in the sky for their sake;
He made for them plants and cattle,
Fowl and fish to feed them.
He slew his foes, reduced his children,
When they thought of making rebellion.
He makes daylight for their sake,
He sails by to see them.
He has built his shrine around them,
When they weep he hears.
He made for them rulers in the egg,
Leaders to raise the back of the weak.
He made for them magic as weapons
To ward off the blow of events,
Guarding, them by day and by night.
He has slain the traitors among them,
As a man beats his son for his brother's sake,
For God knows every name.

(32) Do not neglect my speech,
Which lays down all the laws of kingship,
Which instructs you, that you may rule the land,
And may you reach me with none to accuse you!
Do not kill one who is close to you,
Whom you have favored, God knows him;
He is one of the fortunate ones on earth,
Divine are they who follow the king!
Make yourself loved by everyone,
A good character is remembered [when his time] has passed.
May you be called "he who ended the time of trouble,"
By those who come after in the House of Khety,
In thinking of what has come today.
Lo, I have told you the best of my thoughts,
Act by what is set before you!

The Ancient Egyptian Wisdom Texts

Commentary by Muata Ashby

The Instructions To Merikara

The numbered paragraphs below correspond to the numbered paragraphs in the Merikara writings.

1- The Teachings to Merikara open with a declaration that a person who is "hot-headed" incites people. This is easily noted in human nature in people who are constantly argumentative and always seeking to stir up trouble. Why is this? These people have a deep rooted feeling of discontent which they constantly strive to fill. Not knowing any better way to stop their feeling of inner sorrow, frustration and disappointment, they make others miserable and stir up trouble everywhere, thinking that somehow they are attacking the source of their troubles. They feel satisfied when others are agitated although this is short lived. This is because the true source of their troubles is their inability to understand and cope with their desires. Ignorant of their Divine essence people seek fulfillment through worldly activities and through worldly means. This inevitably leads to frustration and sorrow. When people act out of sorrow, scorn and malice, in reality it is an expression of their pain and ignorance.

2- From a practical perspective a person who lives by unrighteousness should be denounced to the authorities. Society cannot exist in harmony if unrighteousness is allowed to move freely and is unchallenged.

The Ancient Egyptian Wisdom Texts

3- "Good Nature" or virtuous character in a human being is what allows a person to experience the Divine. How is this possible? Every human being is composed of a body and soul. The soul is pure, immortal and without malice. However, when the soul associates itself with matter (a human body) in order to acquire human experiences, it forgets its Divine origin and falls under the clutches of ignorance and human desires. These desires lead to feelings of frustration, anger, hatred, greed and so on. These in turn agitate the mental nature to such a degree that the Divine feeling remains far away. Spiritual practice entails regaining the Divine feeling by cultivating good nature in the human heart. This will become clearer as we move along.

4- Most people believe that physical might is more important than moral force. When a person uses physical violence it is an expression of their lack of patience and mental strength. The practice of non-violence requires great strength and patience. In the end, it overcomes physical might because moral righteousness is based on truth and truth is an eternal reality and carries a Divine sanction. Physical might is a transient phenomena of the material world used by the human ego in order to gain a particular objective in the hope of achieving egoistic fulfillment. However, since true, abiding fulfillment is not possible in the world of time and space, those who use physical violence will never discover peace.

5- One who studies the teachings (Wisdom of Mystical Spirituality) develops subtlety of intellect. He or she gains the ability to control the mind and to understand the desires of the heart. They can rise above the pettiness of egoism and thereby control others who are being led by their egoistic desires since those desires are clouding their intellectual ability. Thus, a learned one is a storehouse of knowledge for all. The teachings are to be studied, copied and internalized within the heart. Subtlety of intellect allows a Sage to cut through the noise of desires in the mind in order to immediately reveal the truth in any situation. There are no illusions in the heart of a Sage. Therefore, only truth can exist. In the heart of a passionate person the truth is seen according to the desires and that person pursues a course which will fulfill the desires. However this is a road leading to disappointment and frustration.

8- The masses value fame and fortune; so much so sometimes that they do things which are unrighteous in order to receive accolades and praises. They are always concerned about what others think of them and there is a constant fear of gossip. They maintain a private set of moral standards and a public set. This two-faced way of life is full of tension and stress and eventually leads to their public ruin.

9- The path of Osiris is the path of righteousness ant Truth. Those who live according to the precepts of Maat are allowed to move forward on the spiritual journey while those who lead a life based on vice and untruth, i.e. those who indulge themselves in human pleasures and desires and do not restrain themselves, are left behind. This implies a movement towards either enlightenment or a movement towards reincarnation and the cycle of birth and death wherein the soul experiences being born, growing up and dying over and over again.

The Ancient Egyptian Wisdom Texts

10- The importance of good association is being alluded to here. It is important to have good council because life has many possibilities for either situations which lead to happiness or situations which lead to sorrow and frustration. Therefore, true riches should be measured in one's noble (righteous) acquaintances rather than material wealth because those values are perishable and fraught with worldly entanglements, which agitate the mind, and draw one into conflict and delusion.

11, 12- There should not be a difference between one's home (private) life and one's public life. There should be truth in all situations of life. One who is truthful engenders respect in all. Unrighteous activities evoke feelings of disrespect and hatred from others.

13- Even though the evil of an evildoer seems to go unpunished, God is the ever-present reality who is aware of every activity and every thought. This is because the human soul is intimately related to God. It is the very expression of the Divine. Thus, nothing can escape God's awareness. Most human beings believe themselves to be separate and distinct from God. In reality this feeling of separation is based on ignorance and illusion. The ignorance and illusion is sustained by the mental agitation. However, when peace, harmony and wisdom are cultivated, spiritual sensitivity is discovered. This is why the wisdom teachings again and again emphasize the need for developing contentment, peace of mind and righteousness. In righteousness there is no agitation, tension or stress because when you live for righteousness sake you are drawing a Divine nectar of Divine feeling. Truth and God are synonymous, therefore,

The Ancient Egyptian Wisdom Texts

living upon truth is in effect living on God. It is this movement which leads to true fulfillment of the needs of the soul which no worldly activity or object of possession can come close to. This section also implies that there is a big difference between someone who has "chanted the writings" and who "strode freely in the secret place" as opposed to someone who has not. This is an allusion to the study of the mystical wisdom teachings and the practice of the rituals in the Ancient Egyptian Temple. One who has begun to study and practice the teachings is special because spiritual aspiration is a rare occurrence in human life. Once a person truly realizes that there is something other than the phenomenal world of time and space he or she begins to search for answers to transcendental questions like "Who am I? What is my purpose? Is there a God? How am I related to God? etc. This sets them apart from the masses who are only concerned with getting ahead in life from a worldly point of view. They are not interested in the mystical wisdom teachings of (mysteries of the temple-Yoga philosophy) but rather with acquiring material wealth and with experiencing the pleasures of the senses. The mass mentality is based on limitation and ignorance because sense pleasures are fleeting while spiritual realization is abiding and leads to immortality and supreme bliss. True happiness is when the soul (*ba*) "comes to the place it knows." This means that it settles to the place of peace and true happiness. Most people are constantly searching for happiness through worldly means. The soul is never satisfied with these and is constantly agitated, moving, searching, etc. However, when spiritual studies and spiritual practice is engaged in, the soul comes to the place it truly knows. The practice of the teachings, prayer, righteous action (virtuous living), chanting the writings, etc. all constitute the process of giving water to the *ba*.

14- This passage is of extreme importance to the understanding of mystical philosophy and it is artistically written so as to convey many powerful teachings in a condensed form. The teacher emphasizes the importance of performing righteous actions in this lifetime because he will be judged by the assessors of MAAT who exist in a different time reference than the one which is known by ordinary humans. Thus, in the ancient times we find teachings in reference to the relativity of time and of Karma (Egyptian-Meskhenet or Meskhen). As a spiritual aspirant, a person is to develop a keen understanding of the relativity of time. In reality, there is no time, only eternity. Out of this eternity, the human mind has recognized elements which it calls events and has created a concept of time in which those events "take place." However, the Ancient Egyptian teachings of Creation teach that there are three main realms of existence, Physical, Astral and Causal. These three realms contain their own apparent realities and their own apparent passage of time which is relative to the others. A human being also has three levels of conscious experience. This is why a human being experiences the passage of time differently when in different states of mind. When you are dreaming you experience a certain passage of time. When you are awake you experience a certain passage of time. When you are asleep but not dreaming you experience a certain passage of time. All these experiences are distinct from the others and seem real within their own experience, so which is the real one? Think of eternity as an endless flow of water in a river. Time is like taking a glass and scooping out one drop of that river and living an entire lifetime within that drop. When human life is beset by ignorance, there is only awareness of the drop. However, when spiritual wisdom is experienced through the practices of yoga, it is possible to discover the eternal nature of existence, one's own immortality and divinity. Thus, time is illusory and only has validity in the relative world of human experience. When enlightenment dawns on the mind, the absolute, eternal and transcendental nature of existence becomes revealed in a flash of a moment. Therefore, as a spiritual aspirant, your goal is to develop a keen understanding and discernment between the relative or practical realities to which the mind and body are bound and transcendental nature of the Self within.

15- When living in society and occupying a position of leadership it is important to raise one's offspring or the youth one is responsible for with the teachings of righteousness and with good will. It is important to give abundantly according to one's means and not to hoard one's possessions or wealth. Hoarding promotes jealousy in others but more importantly it creates an obstruction to one's ability to care for others. This is because ones primary preoccupation is with acquiring wealth and property and finding ways to protect it from others instead of thinking of ways in which to help people and provide for their welfare. Amassing material wealth and the preoccupation with possessions is the mentality of the masses. Objects do not last even when acquired righteously. Further, they cannot bring happiness or true security. Even the richest person can be swallowed up in an earthquake and what good would all the riches in the world do for that person? As we will see, true security and happiness comes from reliance on *Pa*

The Ancient Egyptian Wisdom Texts

Neter, The God, and not on material wealth.

16- This hekau contains a profound teaching of mystical spirituality. It teaches the need to maintain equal vision or equanimity of mind. Since material wealth is transient and illusory as we saw in the last passage, a person cannot be judged by his or her material condition. Rather, a person should be judged for their actions and abilities. Since every human being is innately a Divine, immortal soul, their potential is limitless. What holds people back is their ignorant understanding of life and egoistic feelings which lead to sinful behaviors (behaviors based on vices). If you judge others based on their level of material wealth you are engaging in sin because you are seeing them through your egoistic vision of what is true and real based on ignorance. Virtue is the only true wealth and it expresses in the form of compassion, non-violence, truth, universal love, harmony, sharing, etc. Virtue is an expression of ones understanding of the interconnectedness of life and one's own transcendental existence which is connected to the Supreme Spirit. To the extent that one is aware of one's own Divine nature virtue manifests through the human personality. To the extent that one is in ignorance about one's own Divine nature, sinful (vice) behavior based on greed, jealousy, egoistic desires, etc. will manifest.

17- This hekau refers to material values versus spiritual values of life. Most people are so caught up in the rat race of life and the competition for acquiring success in the world that they neglect spirituality. Spiritual practice or Yoga, is any activity which serves to bring a person closer to Divine awareness. The goal of yoga and mystical spirituality is to

The Ancient Egyptian Wisdom Texts

promote integration of the mind-body-spirit complex in order to produce optimal health of the human being. This is accomplished through mental and physical exercises which promote the free flow of spiritual energy by reducing mental complexes caused by ignorance. There are two roads which human beings can follow, one of wisdom and the other of ignorance. The path of the masses is generally the path of ignorance which leads them into negative situations, thoughts and deeds. These in turn lead to ill health and sorrow in life. The other road is based on wisdom and it leads to health, true happiness and enlightenment. In Ancient Egypt one of the most popular forms of spiritual practice was the ritual worship and Identification with the Divine. Rituals are a powerful method of engendering a spiritual feeling and for increasing spiritual knowledge. Religion in its complete form has three levels. These are *Myth, Ritual* and *Metaphysics* or *Mystical Philosophy.* If religion is not practiced in its entirety there will be a misunderstood movement in spirituality. At the level of myths and rituals all religions of the world appear to be different. However, at the level of mysticism all religious philosophies are aiming for the same goal, to discover the truth about the universe and of the human heart. Thus as a person lives in the world of human experience and strives for success he or she should also engage in daily spiritual practices which will lead to upliftment and which will give direction to life based on sublime goals and aspirations. The ultimate and most sublime goal of life is to discover God and to unite with God. Therefore, all activities in life should be pursued with this goal in mind, making sure that one's actions are not leading one astray through, ignorance, overindulgence and vice. Also you must realize that life is constantly pressuring you and providing you with messages. Advertisements, people and your own desires are constantly whispering in your mind and urging you to act one way or another, to feel one way or another. Daily spiritual practice allows you to receive an uplifting message which will lead you through the forest of decisions, troubles of life. Those who do not engage in daily spiritual practice are as if alone in the world. They are at the mercy of life's situations without a higher vision of life. It must be clearly understood that spiritual practice here implies the process of studying, practicing and meditating upon the teachings under the guidance of an authentic Spiritual Preceptor. Many people feel that going to church once a week or reading a spiritual text will lead them to spiritual enlightenment. This idea is limited and will lead to misunderstanding and frustration. (See the book *Initiation Into Egyptian Yoga* for more on the daily spiritual practices.)

23- This hekau extols the virtue of giving to others and not depriving them. When there is need in a persons heart it has a way of causing stress and even despair. People can be inspired to greatness with goodness rather than with harshness. When people are inspired by sublime goals and led by those who are righteous it will engender in them a feeling of righteousness and solidarity. When people work together there is harmony and harmony translates into prosperity and more good feeling. *Hapy* is the neter who represents the Nile, especially when in flood. The Nile river floods its banks and in so doing brings nutrients and water to the crops which line the banks. Therefore, Hapy represents prosperity and abundance. Neters are normally understood as gods and goddesses who emanate from the Supreme Being, *Pa Neter,* The God. However, neters should be as well understood as cosmic forces which emanate from the Supreme Being and through which the Supreme

Being sustains Creation. Thus, the neters permeate Creation as well as every human being. The neters are the source of life.

24- In the book, *Egyptian Yoga: The Philosophy of Enlightenment*, the teaching of hekau 24 was introduced. Beware of your environment. Beware of your surroundings. Harshness in the surroundings and general environment can cause negative stress which could lead to an unsettled mind.

An unsettled mind is difficult to control. A mind that is uncontrollable will have difficulty in concentrating. Poor concentration will not allow for reflection. Reflection is necessary to make sense of one's situation and to gain intellectual understanding. A non-reflective, confused or "Wrong thinking" mind will have difficulty meditating.

A non-meditating mind will have difficulty in transcending the world of apparent dualities. One will be endlessly pulled into the "world" and the apparent thoughts going on in the mind.

As the mind will be caught up in the endless waves of joys and sorrows, it will be unable to find peace. A mind filled with too much joy or too much sorrow due to its experiences in the world will be equally agitated and one will have difficulty concentrating and calming down. One extreme (ex. Joy) leads to another (ex. Pain).

The concept of the *"Miserable Asiatic"* was also known in Egypt as the concept of *"The Land of Heru and the Land of Set."* Since Set is the God of the desert, the Asiatics, who dwelt in the desert lands, became identified with Set and therefore,

The Ancient Egyptian Wisdom Texts

Setian behavior (impulsive, selfish, brute force, etc.). The teaching about the miserable Asiatic is of paramount importance because it provides an understanding of how the human mind becomes degraded and violent. A human being who is not nurtured and who is constantly experiencing stress due to lack of security, not knowing where the next meal is coming from, how to acquire the acquire and secure the needs of life and then how to hold onto them, etc. All of these worries cause a degradation in the human mind wherein the concern is not with working with others but with competing with them for food, material wealth, mates, etc. The purpose of human existence is to provide a means for the soul to experience and grow in awareness of itself as one with Creation. This feeling is blissful, supremely satisfying and universal. When the soul in a human being is not allowed to express itself in this manner the ego in a human being is in control and this egoism fosters feelings of personal desire, separation, animosity to anything which prevents the ego from getting what it wants. This is the source of animosity, enmity, anger, hatred and violence in human experience. Spiritual practice leads a human being to discover a deeper essence of life. True spiritual understanding allows a person to understand where true happiness and peace are to be found. It shows a person that security cannot be found in the world but in that which sustains it.

27-Ancient Egypt suffered many invasions from Asia. Asia includes Greece, Rome, and the land today known as the "Middle East." Over a period of thousands of years the Asiatics tried to conquer Egypt and through their contact with them the Ancient Egyptians realized the cause of negativity in the heart of the Asiatic peoples. The disposition toward destruction and causing misery to others is a demoniac quality which must be confronted by those who are righteous. This is one of the reasons why several Ancient Egyptian rulers sought to conquer Asia in order to civilize it and thus secure Egypt from outside attacks as well as to provide the Asiatic peoples with a higher vision of life. It is written that Osiris and later Ramses II stretched the borders of Egypt to as far as India and Southern Europe. This passage also includes another important teaching in reference to the fate of those who engage in sin and negativity. The "rebel" (unrighteous person) will be overcome by God. At the time of the judgment of a person's actions a person reaps the reward for his or her deeds. A righteous person should therefore stand up to unrighteousness first by being an example of righteousness and then by pointing out unrighteousness. Moral correctness is stronger than physical might and for this reason any and all forms of unrighteousness can be overcome by perfection in righteousness. A righteous person should not engage in procrastination, delay, excuses, etc. when it comes to asserting the truth even when it means that one's ego will be hurt. One can exercise compassion when telling others of their own mistakes but one should not allow even a small mistake of one's own to go unnoticed. For example if an acquaintance is not ready to hear a criticism of their actions you may withhold the truth until the person is ready to hear it unless they are in imminent danger. One should not tell the truth indiscriminately if it will only serve to hurt people. This would be an expression of one's own ego.

28- One who has real knowledge, that which comes from spiritual experience, becomes the ruler of the Higher Self and the lower nature. The way to achieve this is to have proper guidance and good associations. This means keeping company with virtuous personalities and those who are wise. Once again the

The Ancient Egyptian Wisdom Texts

importance of acting righteously is mentioned. Along with this it is important to be vigilant not only in ones job or career but in one's mind. How often does the mind stray into thoughts of negativity (anger, depression, hatred, etc.) and how often are these stray thoughts checked before they enter deep into the heart and engender negative activities? A spiritual aspirant must develop vigilance in every aspect of life so as not to allow unrighteousness in their environment which they have the power to control or prevent. At the end of this hekau the injunction of karma, which is well known in modern times as "What you do comes back to you." Also, this teaching expresses very succinctly a knowledge of the principles which govern creation. These were expressed thousands of years later by Sir Isaac Newton in his Principia (1687) as three laws of motion. These laws form the basis of the classical study of force and motion. According to the Third Law, to every action there is an equal and opposite reaction. While Mr. Newton was referring primarily to nature and matter in particular, the Ancient Egyptian reference relates also to human nature and the laws of karmic interrelationships in society as well as in nature.

29- This hekau is very insightful because it shows, in very brief statements, that God, who is variously known as "the Hidden One" or *Shetai,* is the knower of the character of human beings. God is the innermost essence of every human being. Therefore, God is the eternal witness to every thought, feeling or desire which enters the mind. Thus God "knows" all characters. God is also all-encompassing and therefore all that can be detected with the human senses is endowed with God's presence.

30- Just as the bed or channel of a waterway brings water to one destination and having reached there the water takes on a new course in a different channel or waterway, so to the nature as an expression of the Self is ever flowing and relentlessly moving toward the ocean. So too the Soul (ba) is relentlessly moving through many incarnations in a search for its true abode. Thus, it is important to worship the Self (God) in all forms in Creation or expressions as one moves through the paths of life. This worship will ultimately lead to self discovery and spiritual enlightenment. This implies acting in accordance with Maat (truth, righteousness, etc.) and also this implies selfless service to humanity and to nature. God and Creation are synonymous. Therefore, if you truly propose to work for God you must understand that God is expressing as the needy, the sick, the homeless, the depressed, etc. Thus, you must render service by doing what you can to alleviate suffering in the world and to promote harmony and goodwill. All creatures on earth and in the universe are your kin and should be treated as sacred beings, no matter how low they have come to be or how high they may appear. This way of life will purify your heart and allow you to see through the pettiness and pathetic aspect of human egoism and ignorance. The final statement of this hekau emphatically states that living according to this understanding will allow a person to draw Divine Grace. Divine Grace is spiritual wealth in the form of greater inner peace, contentment, wisdom, health, happiness and the unfoldment of the inner gifts of the soul. This is the basis for the wondrous acts which have been performed by Saints and Sages throughout the ages.

31- Indeed Creation has only one purpose, to create experiences for human consciousness and to promote the evolution of the Soul. God, the Self, is behind every aspect of creation and the one who has fashioned the elements in such a way that they sustain life. The very life force (breath), which is indispensable to life, is the dynamic essence of the Self. Human beings (male and female alike) are the reflections of God. In fact the entire Creation, nature, animals, plants, the planets and stars are expressions of God in much the same way as an image in a mirror is an expression of the object being reflected. Another example is a dream. When you dream, the dream world is an expression, a reflection of your consciousness. All of the people and places in your dream are an expression of your consciousness. In the same way, Creation is an expression of God's consciousness. Thus, every human being is god or goddess, endowed with the power to create according to the level of attunement with the Cosmic Self. A human being can create a dream world because he or she is empowered with the consciousness of God. When there is negativity and ignorance in the mind the power is reflected in limitation. However, when a human being moves toward spiritual enlightenment the ego-self becomes like a thin mist which allows a person to behold the grandeur of their true Self as one with God. Then the power, which was always there, can be harnessed and used in accordance with the Divine Plan (Maat). In reality there is no separation between human beings and God. This is the greatest teaching of this text. Every human being emanated from God's body as it were, as a thought emanates from the mind and all Creation is God's body. This teaching was the resounding theme of Theban and Memphite Theology in Ancient Egypt. However, due to ignorance and externalization, the human personality cannot see the glory of its origin and true Self. Thus, spiritual disciplines such as the various Yoga disciplines as well as the religions which have developed over time, exist with the sole purpose of reuniting a human being, endowed with an individual, limited Soul with God, the Universal Soul.

The Ancient Egyptian Wisdom Texts

32- In the Bible book of *Matthew 5:9* says *"Blessed [are] the peacemakers: for they shall be called children of God"* —Jesus

In the Christian Bible Jesus instructs his disciples in what are today regarded as beatitudes, or conduct which leads to blessedness (spiritual evolution and peace). This teaching was given thousands of years before in the teachings to Merikara (May you be called "he who ended the time of trouble.") The peacemaker is one who understands the harmony which underlies the apparent chaos of nature and who also understands human nature. In ignorance people fight amongst themselves as animals. One who is growing in knowledge will be free of egoism and will thus be able to act on necessity and righteousness rather than on egoistic desires and impulses of the lower nature. Being a peacemaker implies being an example of peacefulness for society as well as a teacher of righteousness and a promoter of good will. Therefore there is an exhortation in the final section that this teaching needs to be followed and practiced in order for it to become effective. Intellectual knowledge without practice is like placing food on a plate with all of the necessary condiments but without eating it and assimilating it. Wisdom is not something that occurs by magic or chance. It is a process of inner growth through knowledge and experience. Thus the Wisdom Texts impart the understanding that Action, the path of Maat, leads to purification and spiritual enlightenment.

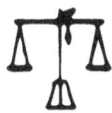

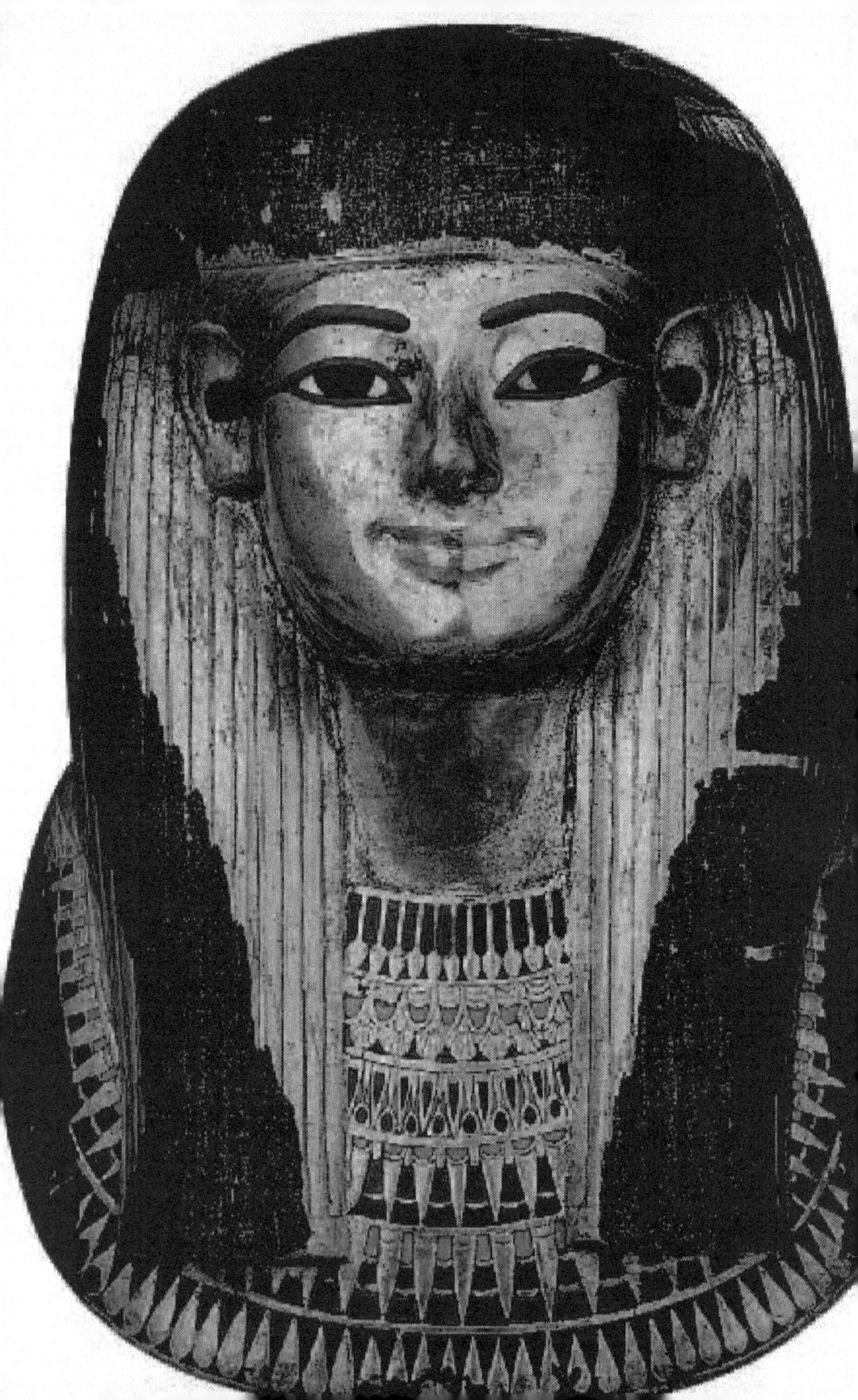

The Ancient Egyptian Wisdom Texts

The Teachings of Sehtpabri

This poem to King Amenemhēt III (1844–1797 B.C.) is included in this section, because its author claims to have composed it for the instruction of his children. He was a high official in the treasury, and must also have been brought into personal contact with the king, for he speaks of himself as " one whom his lord exalted in front of millions, a real confidant of his lord, to whom hidden things were spoken." He, moreover, proclaims this close connection with his lord by placing—against all precedent—the following verses on his tomb-stone,² which he scholastically designates his " Instruction."

Instruction which he composed for his children.

I tell of a great matter and cause you to hear (it). I impart to you a thought for eternity, and a maxim for right living (?) ³ and for the spending of a lifetime in bliss.

Revere King Nemaatrē, who ever liveth, in your bodies, and consort with his majesty in your hearts.

He is Understanding, which is in the hearts, and his eyes search out every body. He is Rē, by whose rays men see.

He illumineth the Two Lands more than the sun. He maketh the Two Lands more verdant than doth a high Nile. He hath filled the Two Lands with strength and life.

The nostrils become cool when he inclineth to terror.⁴ When he is gracious, then (?) men breathe the air.

He giveth vital force to them that serve him, he supplieth food to them that tread his path. The king is Vital Force and his mouth ⁵ Abundance.

¹ *I.e.* probably : Do not make away with your kinsmen on coming to the throne—as so often is done in the East.

² Cairo 20538. The quite obvious stanzas should be noted.

³ A special device has been employed here by the poet. Not only do the three words " for right living " form a pun on the immediately following name of his king, but he has contrived so to arrange the signs that they look like this name.

⁴ Meaning ?

⁵ Which utters his commands. The passage merely states that the king sees that his faithful subjects are provided for.

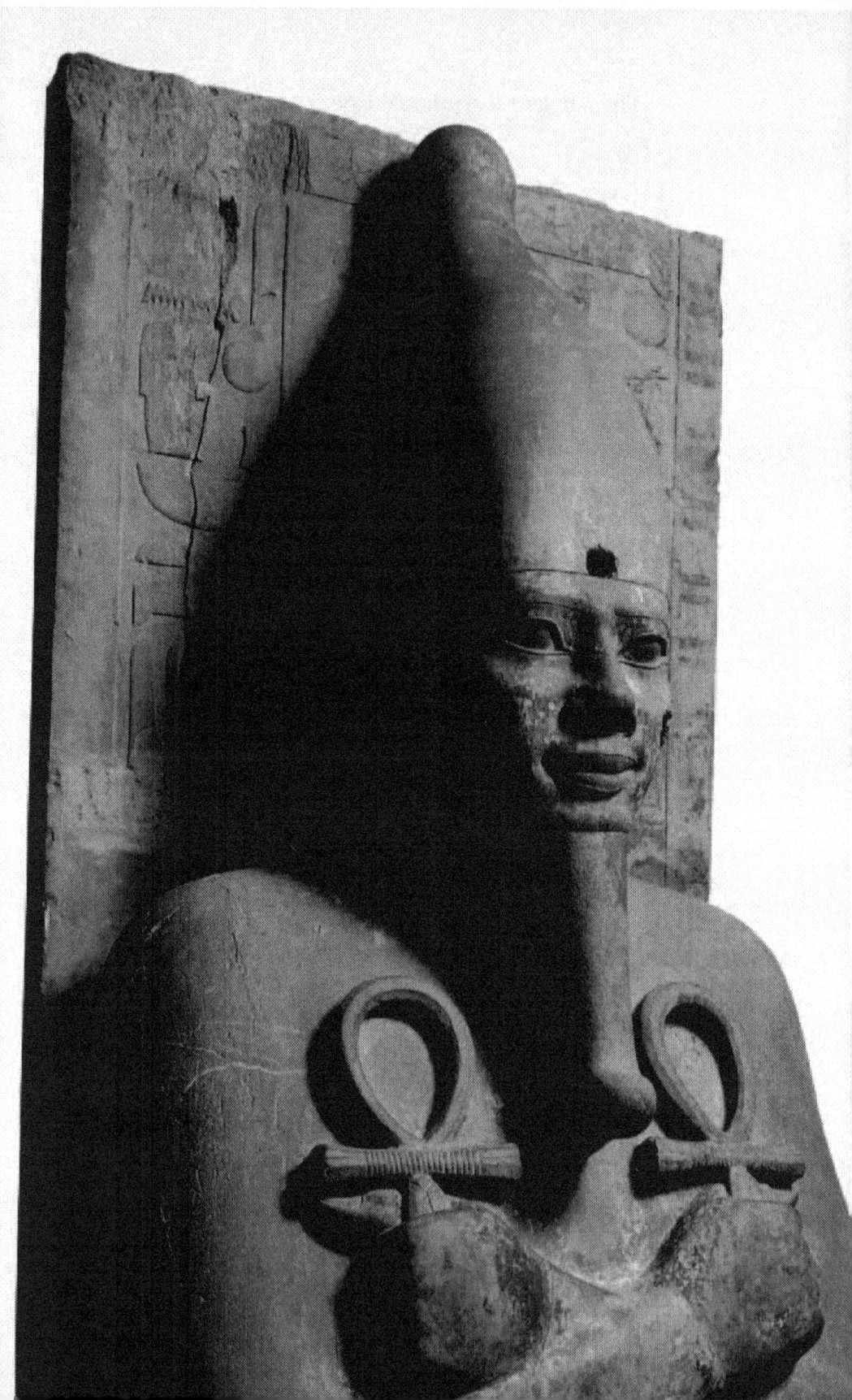

The Ancient Egyptian Wisdom Texts

THE INSTRUCTION OF AMENEMOPE

Introduction

(i) Beginning of the teaching for life,
The instructions for well-being,
Every rule for relations with elders,
For conduct toward magistrates;
Knowing how to answer one who speaks,
To reply to one who sends a message.
So as to direct him on the paths of life,
To make him prosper upon earth;
To let his heart enter its shrine,
Steering clear of evil;
To save him from the mouth of strangers,
To let (him) be praised in the mouth of people. Made by the overseer of fields, experienced in his office,

He says:

Chapter I

(1) Give your ears, hear the sayings,
Give your heart to understand them;
It is an advantage to put them in your heart,
If you neglect them you will suffer!
Let them rest in the container of your belly,
May they be bolted in your heart;
(2) When there rises a whirlwind of words,
They'll be a mooring post for your tongue,
a guide.
If you make your life with these in your heart, You will find it success and safety;
You will find my words a storehouse for life, Your being will prosper while upon earth.

Chapter 2

(3) Beware of robbing a wretch,
Of attacking a cripple;

The Ancient Egyptian Wisdom Texts

Don't stretch out your hand to touch an old man, Nor [speak harshly] to an elder.
Don't let yourself be sent on a mischievous errand,
Nor be friends with him who does it.

(3)   Don't create a disturbance or an outburst against the one who attacks you,
Also, do not answer him or attack him yourself.
Whoever does evil will be rejected by the shore,
Its floodwater carries them away.
The northwind comes to stop their unrighteousness,
(4)   It mixes with the thunderstorm.
The storm cloud is large, and the crocodiles are vicious,
You heated man, how are you now?
He cries out, and his voice reaches the heavens,
But it is the Moon who declares his crime.
(5)   Steer, we will ferry the wicked,
We do not act like his kind;
Lift him up, give him your hand,
Leave him (in) the hands of The God;

(6)   Fill his belly with bread of your own give him drink, for it is in the heart of the God to show another act of compassion,
That he be sated and weep.
Another thing good in the heart of The God:
To pause before speaking.

Chapter 3

(7)   Don't start a quarrel with a hot-mouthed man,
Nor needle him with words.
Pause before a foe, bend before an attacker, Sleep (meditate on it) before speaking.
A storm that bursts like fire in straw,
(8)   Such is, the heated man in his hour.
Withdraw from him, leave him alone,
The God knows how to answer him.
If you Make your life with these (words) in your heart,
Your children will observe them.

The Ancient Egyptian Wisdom Texts

Chapter 4

(9) As for the heated man in the temple,
He is like a tree growing [indoors];
A moment lasts its growth of [shoots]
Its end comes about in the woodshed;
(10)   It is floated far from its place,
The flame is its burial shroud.
The truly silent, who keeps apart,
He is like a tree grown in a meadow.
It greens, it doubles its yield,
(11)   It stands in front, of its lord.
Its fruit is sweet, its shade delightful,
Its end comes in the garden.

Chapter 5

(12) Do not falsify the temple rations,
Do not be greedy and you'll find profit.
Do not remove a servant of The God,
So as to do favors to another.
(13) Do not say: "Today is like tomorrow, How will this end?
(14) Comes tomorrow, today has vanished,
The deep has become the water's edge. Crocodiles are bared, hippopotami stranded, The fish crowded together .
(15)   Jackals are sated, birds are in feast,
The fishnets have been drained.
But all the silent in the temple,
They say: "Ra's blessing is great."
Cling to the silent, then you find life,
(16) Your being will prosper upon earth.

Chapter 6

(17)   Do not move the markers on the borders of fields,
Nor shift the position of the measuring-cord.
Do not be greedy for a cubit of land,
(18) Nor encroach on the boundaries of a widow.
The trodden path worn down by time,
He who disguises it in the fields,
When he has snared (it) by false oaths,
(19) He will be caught by the might of the Moon.

The Ancient Egyptian Wisdom Texts

Recognize him who does this on earth: He is an oppressor of the weak,
A foe bent on destroying your being,
The taking of life is in his eye.
(20)   His house is an enemy to the town,
His storage bins will be destroyed;
His wealth will be seized from his children's hands,
His possessions will be given to another.
Beware of destroying the borders of fields,
(21)   Lest a terror carry you away;
One pleases God with the might of the lord
When one discerns the borders of fields.
Desire your being to be sound,
Beware of Neberdjer, the Lord of All;
(22)   Do not erase another's marker,
It profits you to keep it sound.
Plow your fields and you'll find what you need, You'll receive bread from your threshing-floor.
(23)   Better is a bushel given you by The God,
Than thousands through wrongdoing.
Pass not thy day in beer-houses and eating or thou wilt become a mere mass of food.
The beggar in God's hand is better off than the rich man in his palace. Crusts of bread and a loving heart are better than rich food and mental unrest. Hanker not after dainty Mind thy business, and let every man do his when he wishes to do it. Learn to be content with what thou hast.
Possessions and wealth gained wrongly stay not a day in bin and barn,
They make no food for the beer jar;
A moment is their stay in the granary,
If thou sailest with a thief thou wilt be left in the river.
(24)   Better is poverty in the hand of The God, Than -wealth in the storehouse;
Better is bread with a happy heart ,
Than wealth with vexation.

Chapter 7

(25) Do not set your heart on wealth,
There is no ignoring Fate and Destiny;
Do not let your heart go straying,
Every man comes to his hour.
Do not strain to seek increase,
(26) What you have, let it suffice you.

The Ancient Egyptian Wisdom Texts

If riches come to you by theft,
They will not stay the night with you.
Comes day they are not in your house,
Their place is seen but they are not there;
(27)   Earth opened its mouth, leveled them, swallowed them,
And made them sink into dat.
They made a hole as big as their size,
And sank into the Netherworld;
They made themselves wings like geese,
And flew away to the sky.
(28)   Do not rejoice in wealth from theft,
Nor complain of being poor.
If the leading archer presses forward,
His company abandons him;
(29) The boat of the greedy is left (in) the mud,
While the bark of the silent sails with the wind. Get into the habit of praying sincerely to Aten (i.e. the solar Disk) as he rises in the sky, saying,

Saying: "Grant me strength, well-being and health";
He will give you your needs for this life,
And you will be safe from fear.

Chapter 8

(30)   Set your goodness before people,
Then you are greeted by all;
One welcomes the Uraeus, Approve what is good,
Spits upon Apopis, what is bad.
(31) Guard your tongue from harmful speech,
Then you will be loved by others.
You will find your place in the Sanctuary, the house of God, Be kind to the poor. Get thee a seat in the sanctuary. Be strong to do the Will of God.
You will share in the offerings of your lord.
(32)   When you're revered and your coffin conceals you,
You will be safe through the power of God."
(33) Do not shout "crime" against a man,
When the cause of (his) flight is hidden. Hide the flight of the runaway slave.
(34) Whether you hear something good or evil,
Do it outside where it is not heard.
Disregard what thou hearest, whether good or bad; it is not thy business, heed it not. Speak only what is good, what is bad hide in thy belly.

The Ancient Egyptian Wisdom Texts

Chapter 9

(35)   Do not befriend the heated man,
Nor approach him for conversation. Avoid the scandal-monger.
His lips are datesyrup, his tongue is a deadly dagger, and a blazing fire is within him. Avoid converse with evil men, for that God hates. Make thy plans wisely. Be dignified. Place thyself for safety in the hand of God. The liar is an abomination to him.
(36)   Keep your tongue from answering your superior,
And take care not to insult him.
Let him not cast his speech to catch you,
Nor give free rein to your answer.
Converse with a man of your own measure,
And take care not to [offend] him.
(37)   Swift is the speech of one who is angered,
More than wind [over] water.
He tears down, he builds up with his tongue, When he makes his hurtful speech.
(38)   He gives an, answer worthy of a beating,
For its weight is harm.
He hauls freight like all the world,
But his load is falsehood.
He is the ferryman of snaring words,
He goes and comes with quarrels.
When he eats and drinks inside,
His answer is (heard) outside.
(39) The day he is charged with his (Angry person, angry speech) crime
Is misfortune for his children.
If only Khnum (Knum) came to him,
The Potter to the heated man,
So as to knead the [defect in the] heart.
He is like a young wolf in the farmyard,
He turns one eye against the other,
He causes brothers to quarrel.
He runs before every wind like clouds,
He dims the radiance of the sun;
He flips his tail like the crocodile's young,
His lips are sweet, his tongue is bitter,
A fire burns in his belly.
Don't leap to join such a one,
Lest a terror carry you away.

The Ancient Egyptian Wisdom Texts

Chapter 10

(40)   Don't force yourself to greet the heated man,
For then you injure your own heart;
Do not say "greetings" to him falsely,
While there is terror in your belly.
(41)   Do not speak falsely to a man,
The God, abhors it;
Do not sever your heart from your tongue,
That all your strivings may succeed.
You will be weighty before the others,
And secure in the hand of The God.
God hates the falsifier of words,
He greatly abhors the dissembler

Chapter 11

(42)   Do not covet a poor man's goods,
Nor hunger for his bread;
A poor man's goods are a block in the throat,
It makes the gullet vomit.
He who makes gain by lying oaths,
His heart is misled by his belly;
Where there is fraud success is feeble,
The bad spoils the good.
You will be guilty before your superior,
And confused in your account;
Your pleas will be answered by a curse,
Your prostration's by a beating.
The big mouthful of bread-you swallow, you vomit it,
And you are emptied of your gain.
(43)   Observe the overseer of the poor,
When the stick attains him,
All his people are bound in chains,
And he is led to the executioner.
If you are released, before your superior,
You are yet hateful to your subordinates;
Steer away from the poor man on the road, Look at him and keep clear of his goods.

The Ancient Egyptian Wisdom Texts

Chapter 12

(44)   Do not desire a noble's wealth,
Nor make free with a big mouthful of bread;
If he sets you to manage his property,
Shun his, and yours will prosper.
(45)   Do not converse with a heated man,
So as to befriend a hostile, man.
If you are sent to transport straw,
Stay away from its container.
If a man is observed on a fraudulent errand,
He will not be sent on another occasion.

Chapter 13

(46)   Do not cheat a man (through) pen on scroll,
The God abhors it;
(47)   Do not bear witness with false words,
So as to brush aside a man by your tongue.
(48)   Do not assess a man who has nothing,
And thus falsify your pen.
If you find a large debt against a poor man, Make it into three parts;
Forgive two, let one stand,
(49)   You will find it a path of life.
After sleep, Indulge not in morning slumber whilst the day breaks majestically 'm the sky. What can be compared to dawn and daybreak for beauty ? To what can the man who knows not the dawn be compared? For whilst God is performing His splendid work that man is wallowing in slothfulness.
Better is praise and love of men,
Than material wealth in your storehouse;
Better is bread with a happy heart,
Than wealth with vexation.

Chapter 14

(50) Do not recall yourself to a man,
Nor strain to seek his hand.
If he says to you: "Here is a gift."
[No poor person] will refuse it.
Don't blink at him, nor bow your head,
Nor turn aside your gaze.
Salute him with your mouth, say, "Greetings".

The Ancient Egyptian Wisdom Texts

He will desist and you succeed.
Do not rebuff him in his approach,
[at another time he'll be taken away]

Chapter 15

(51) Do what is good and then you will prosper,
Do not dip your pen to injure a man.
The finger of the scribe is the beak of the Ibis,
Beware of using it wrongly.
(52)   The Ape dwells in the House of Khnum,
His eye encircles the Two Lands;
When he sees one who cheats with his finger,
He carries his livelihood off in the flood.
The scribe who cheats with his finger,
His son will not be enrolled.
(53)   If you make your life with these (words) in your heart,
Your children will observe them.

Chapter 16

(54)   Do not move the scales nor alter the weights,
Nor diminish the fractions o Measure;
(55)   Do not desire a measure of the fields, Nor neglect those of the treasury.
The Ape sits by the balance,
His heart is in the plummet;
Where is a god as great as Djehuti,
Who invented these things and made them?
(56)   Do not make for yourself deficient weights,
(57)   They [the unrighteous liars, schemers, etc] are rich in grief through the might of God.
If you see someone who cheats,
Keep your distance from him.
(58)   Do not covet copper,
Disdain beautiful linen;
What good is one dressed in finery,
If he cheats before The God?.
Faience disguised as gold,
Comes day, it turns to lead.

The Ancient Egyptian Wisdom Texts

Chapter 17

(59) Beware of disguising the measure,
So as to falsify its fractions;
Do not force it to overflow,
Nor let its belly be empty-
Measure according to its true size,
Your hand clearing exactly.
Do not make a bushel of twice its size,
For then you are headed for the abyss.
The bushel is the Eye of Re,
It abhors him who trims;
(60) A measurer who indulges in cheating,
His Eye seals (the verdict) against him.
(61) Do not accept a farmer's dues
And then assess him so as to injure him;
Do not conspire with the measurer,
So as to defraud the share of the Residence. Greater is the might of the threshing floor,
Than an oath by the great throne.

Chapter 18

(62) Do not lie down in fear of tomorrow:
"Comes day, how will tomorrow be?"
Man ignores how tomorrow will be;
God is ever in his perfection,
Man is ever in his failure.
(63) The words men say are one thing,
The deeds of The God are another.
Do not say: "I have done no wrong,"
And then strain to seek a quarrel;
The wrong belongs to The God,
(64) He seals (the verdict) with his finger.
There is no perfection before The God,
But there is imperfection, before him;
(65) If one strains to seek perfection,
In a moment he has marred it.
(66) Keep firm your heart, steady your heart,
Say not, Evil should not be permitted to exist there is neither good nor evil in the hand of the God. A man's tongue may be his steersman, but it is Nebertcher who is the pilot. Cause not the giving of a wrong verdict in the Law Courts by hiding the truth. Accept no bribe. Truth is the great

The Ancient Egyptian Wisdom Texts

support of God (or throne-bearer). Seek not to penetrate the Divine Will, for Destiny and Fate are established.
Waste not the early hours of the day in sleep. Haste not to be rich, but be not slothful in thine own interest.

Chapter 19

(67) Do not go to court before an official
In order to falsify your words;
(68) Do not vacillate in your answers,
When your witnesses accuse.
Do not strain (with) oaths by your lord,
(With) speeches at the hearing;
Tell the truth before the official,
(69) Lest he lay a hand on you.
If another day you come before him,
He will incline to all you say;
He will relate your speech to the Council of Thirty,
It will be observed on another occasion.

Chapter 20

(70) Do not confound a man in the law court,
In order to brush aside one who is right.
(71) Do not incline to-the well-dressed man,
And rebuff the one in rags.
(72) Don't accept the gift of a powerful man,
And deprive the weak for his sake.
(73) A great gift of God, is Maat
Given, it is, only to those chosen by God.
(74) The might of those who resemble God,
The poor are saved from their tormentor through it.
(75) Do not make for yourself false documents,
They are a deadly provocation;
They (mean) the great restraining oath,
They, (mean) a hearing by the herald.
(76) Don't falsify the oracles in the scrolls, And thus disturb the plans of God;
(77) Don't use for yourself the might of God, As if there were no Fate and Destiny.
Hand over property to its owners,

The Ancient Egyptian Wisdom Texts

Thus do you seek life for yourself;
Don't raise your desire in their house,
Or your bones belong to the execution-block.

Chapter 21

(78)   Do not say: "Find me a strong superior, For a man in your town has injured me";
Do not say: "Find me a protector,
'For one who hates me has injured me."
(79)   Indeed you do not know the plans of God,
And should not weep for tomorrow;
Settle in the arms of The God,
Your silence will overthrow them (the wrongdoers).
(80)   The crocodile that makes no sound,
Dread of it is ancient.
(81)   Do not empty your belly to everyone, And thus destroy respect of you;
Broadcast not your words to others,
Nor join with one who bares his heart.
(82)   Better is one whose speech is in his belly,
Than he who tells it to cause harm.
(83)   One does not run to reach success,
One does not move to spoil it.

Chapter 22

(84)   Do not provoke your adversary,
So as to (make) him tell his thoughts;
Do not leap to come before him,
When you do not see his doings.
First gain insight from his answer,
Then keep still and you will succeed.
(85)   Leave it to him to empty his belly,
Know how to sleep, he will be found out.
Do not harm him,
(86)   Be wary of him, do not ignore him. Indeed you do not know the plans of God,
And should not weep for tomorrow;
(87)   Settle in the arms of The God,
Your silence will overthrow them.

The Ancient Egyptian Wisdom Texts

Chapter 23

(88)   Do not eat in the presence of an official
And then set your mouth before (him);
If you are sated pretend to chew,
Content yourself with your saliva.
Look at the bowl that is before you,
And let it serve your needs.
An official is great in his office,
As a well is rich in drawings of water.

Chapter 24

(89)   Do not listen to an official's reply indoors
In order to repeat it to another outside.
(90)   Do not let your word be carried outside,
Lest your heart be aggrieved.
(91)   Beware of neglecting the heart of man, it is a gift of God.
(92)   The name of the man at the side of an official should not be known.

Chapter 25

(93)   Do not laugh at a blind man,
Nor tease a dwarf,
Nor cause hardship for the lame.
Don't tease a man who is in the hand of The God,
Nor be angry with him for his failings.
(94)   Man is straw and clay,
The God is his fashioner.
He destroys, He creates daily,
He makes a thousand to be poor by his will,
He makes, a thousand men into rulers,
When he is in his hour of life.
(95)   Happy is the one who reaches the beautiful west,
When they are safe in the hand of The God.

Chapter 26

(96)   Do not sit down in the beer-house
In order to join one greater than you,
Be he a youth who has become great through his office,
Or if he is an elder through his birth.
Befriend a man of your own caliber,

The Ancient Egyptian Wisdom Texts

Ra is helpful from a distance.
(97)   If you see one of a higher position than you outdoors,
Walk behind him respectfully;
Give a hand to an elder sated with beer,
Respect him as his children would.
(98)   The arm is not hurt by being bared,
The back is not broken by bending it.
A man does not lose anything by speaking sweetly,
Nor does he gain anything if his speech is agitated and irate.
(99)   The pilot who is watchful and alert to what is coming,
He will not wreck his boat.

Chapter 27

(100)   Do not revile one who is older than you,
He has seen Ra before you;
(101)   Let there be no reason for him to report you to the Aten at his rising,
Saying: "A youth has reviled an old man."
Very painful before Pre, Is a youth who reviles an elder.
(102)   Let him beat you while your hand is on your chest,
Let him revile you while you are silent;
(103)   If next day you come before him,
He will give you food in plenty.
A dog's food is from its master,
It barks to him who gives it.

Chapter 28

(104)   Do not revile or assail on a widow when you find her in the fields which are not her own,
And then fail to be patient with her reply.
(105)   Do not refuse your oil jar to a stranger, Double it before your brothers.
(106)   God prefers the person who honors the poor, To the one who worships the wealthy.
The love of God is better than the reverence of the nobleman.

The Ancient Egyptian Wisdom Texts

Chapter 29

(106)   Do not prevent people from crossing the river,
If there is room in the ferry.
(107)   When you are given an oar in the midst of the deep,
Bend your arms and take it.
The God will not be offended thereby.
(108)   Don't make yourself a ferry on the river, And then strain to seek its fare;
(109)   Take the fare from him who is wealthy,
And let pass him who is poor.

Chapter 30

(110)   Look to these thirty Precepts which I have laid out for you,
They inform, they educate;
They are the foremost of all books,
(111)   They make the ignorant wise.
If they are read to the ignorant,
He is cleansed through them.
Mature people who read them will surely steer their course by them.
(112)   Immerse yourself in them, study them well, meditate on them, understand them and put them in your heart,
And become a person who expounds them,
One who expounds as a teacher.
The scribe who is skilled in his office,
He is found worthy to be a courtier.

Colophon

That is its end.

Written by Senu, son of the divine father Pemu.

The Ancient Egyptian Wisdom Texts

Song of the Harper

I have heard these songs
which are in the ancient tombs,
which tell of the virtues of life on earth
and make little of life in the Neterchert (cemetery).
Why then do likewise to eternity?
It is a place of justice, without fear,
where uproar is forbidden,
where no one attacks his fellow.
This place has no enemies;
all our relatives have lived in it from time immemorial,
with millions more to come.
It is not possible to linger in Egypt -
no one can escape from going west (end of life- Netherworld).
One's acts on earth are like a dream.
'Welcome safe and sound!'
to who ever arrives in the West.

-Ancient Egyptian Harper's Song

- "The purpose of all human life is to achieve a state of consciousness apart from bodily concerns."
  •

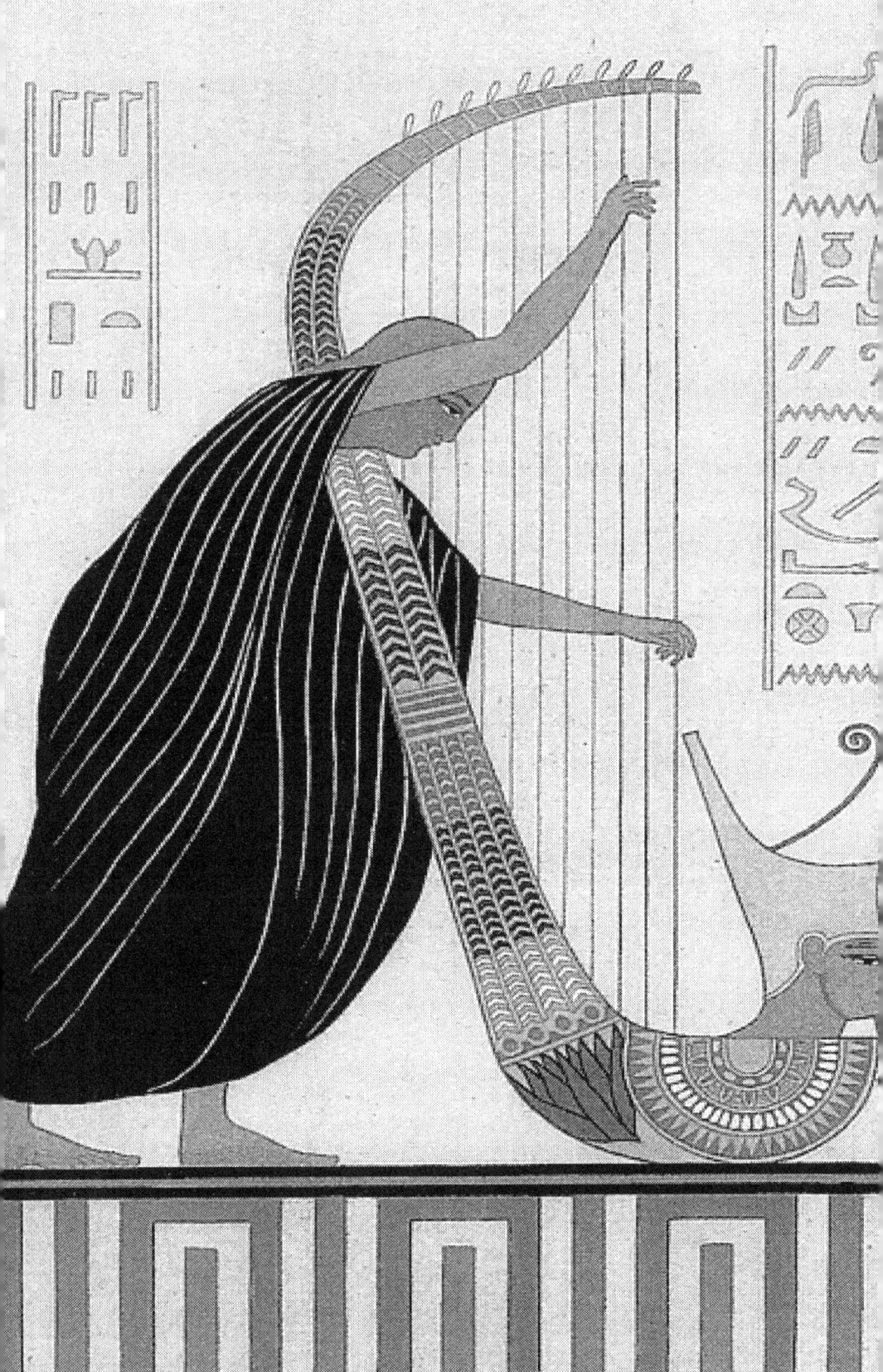

The Ancient Egyptian Wisdom Texts

Other Books From C M Books
P.O.Box 570459
Miami, Florida, 33257
(305) 378-6253 Fax: (305) 378-6253

This book is part of a series on the study and practice of Ancient Egyptian Yoga and Mystical Spirituality based on the writings of Dr. Muata Abhaya Ashby. They are also part of the Egyptian Yoga Course provided by the Sema Institute of Yoga. Below you will find a listing of the other books in this series. For more information send for the Egyptian Yoga Book-Audio-Video Catalog or the Egyptian Yoga Course Catalog.

Now you can study the teachings of Egyptian and Indian Yoga wisdom and Spirituality with the Egyptian Yoga Mystical Spirituality Series. The Egyptian Yoga Series takes you through the Initiation process and lead you to understand the mysteries of the soul and the Divine and to attain the highest goal of life: ENLIGHTENMENT. The *Egyptian Yoga Series*, takes you on an in depth study of Ancient Egyptian mythology and their inner mystical meaning. Each Book is prepared for the serious student of the mystical sciences and provides a study of the teachings along with exercises, assignments and projects to make the teachings understood and effective in real life. The Series is part of the Egyptian Yoga course but may be purchased even if you are not taking the course. The series is ideal for study groups.

Prices subject to change.

1. EGYPTIAN YOGA: THE PHILOSOPHY OF ENLIGHTENMENT An original, fully illustrated work, including hieroglyphs, detailing the meaning of the Egyptian mysteries, tantric yoga, psycho-spiritual and physical exercises. Egyptian Yoga is a guide to the practice of the highest spiritual philosophy which leads to absolute freedom from human misery and to immortality. It is well known by scholars that Egyptian philosophy is the basis of Western and Middle Eastern religious philosophies such as *Christianity, Islam, Judaism,* the *Kabala*, and Greek philosophy, but what about Indian philosophy, Yoga and Taoism? What were the original teachings? How can they be practiced today?

The Ancient Egyptian Wisdom Texts

What is the source of pain and suffering in the world and what is the solution? Discover the deepest mysteries of the mind and universe within and outside of your self. 8.5" X 11" ISBN: 1-884564-01-1 Soft $19.95

2. EGYPTIAN YOGA: African Religion Volume 2- Theban Theology U.S. In this long awaited sequel to *Egyptian Yoga: The Philosophy of Enlightenment* you will take a fascinating and enlightening journey back in time and discover the teachings which constituted the epitome of Ancient Egyptian spiritual wisdom. What are the disciplines which lead to the fulfillment of all desires? Delve into the three states of consciousness (waking, dream and deep sleep) and the fourth state which transcends them all, Neberdjer, "The Absolute." These teachings of the city of Waset (Thebes) were the crowning achievement of the Sages of Ancient Egypt. They establish the standard mystical keys for understanding the profound mystical symbolism of the Triad of human consciousness. ISBN 1-884564-39-9 $23.95

3. THE KEMETIC DIET: GUIDE TO HEALTH, DIET AND FASTING Health issues have always been important to human beings since the beginning of time. The earliest records of history show that the art of healing was held in high esteem since the time of Ancient Egypt. In the early 20th century, medical doctors had almost attained the status of sainthood by the promotion of the idea that they alone were "scientists" while other healing modalities and traditional healers who did not follow the "scientific method' were nothing but superstitious, ignorant charlatans who at best would take the money of their clients and at worst kill them with the unscientific "snake oils" and "irrational theories". In the late 20th century, the failure of the modern medical establishment's ability to lead the general public to good health, promoted the move by many in society towards "alternative medicine". Alternative medicine disciplines are those healing modalities which do not adhere to the philosophy of allopathic medicine. Allopathic medicine is what medical doctors practice by an large. It is the theory that disease is caused by agencies outside the body such as bacteria, viruses or physical means which affect the body. These can therefore be treated by medicines and therapies The natural healing method began in the absence of extensive technologies with the idea that all the answers for health may be found in nature or rather, the deviation from nature. Therefore, the health of the body can be restored by correcting the aberration and thereby restoring balance. This is the area that will be covered in this volume. Allopathic techniques have their place in the art of healing. However, we should not forget that the body is a grand achievement of the spirit and built into it is the capacity to maintain itself and heal itself. Ashby, Muata ISBN: 1-884564-49-6 $28.95

The Ancient Egyptian Wisdom Texts

4. INITIATION INTO EGYPTIAN YOGA Shedy: Spiritual discipline or program, to go deeply into the mysteries, to study the mystery teachings and literature profoundly, to penetrate the mysteries. You will learn about the mysteries of initiation into the teachings and practice of Yoga and how to become an Initiate of the mystical sciences. This insightful manual is the first in a series which introduces you to the goals of daily spiritual and yoga practices: Meditation, Diet, Words of Power and the ancient wisdom teachings. 8.5" X 11" ISBN 1-884564-02-X   Soft Cover $24.95 U.S.

5. *THE AFRICAN ORIGINS OF CIVILIZATION, RELIGION AND YOGA SPIRITUALITY AND ETHICS PHILOSOPHY* HARD COVER EDITION Part 1, Part 2, Part 3 in one volume 683 Pages Hard Cover First Edition Three volumes in one. Over the past several years I have been asked to put together in one volume the most important evidences showing the correlations and common teachings between Kamitan (Ancient Egyptian) culture and religion and that of India. The questions of the history of Ancient Egypt, and the latest archeological evidences showing civilization and culture in Ancient Egypt and its spread to other countries, has intrigued many scholars as well as mystics over the years. Also, the possibility that Ancient Egyptian Priests and Priestesses migrated to Greece, India and other countries to carry on the traditions of the Ancient Egyptian Mysteries, has been speculated over the years as well. In chapter 1 of the book *Egyptian Yoga The Philosophy of Enlightenment,* 1995, I first introduced the deepest comparison between Ancient Egypt and India that had been brought forth up to that time. Now, in the year 2001 this new book, *THE AFRICAN ORIGINS OF CIVILIZATION, MYSTICAL RELIGION AND YOGA PHILOSOPHY,* more fully explores the motifs, symbols and philosophical correlations between Ancient Egyptian and Indian mysticism and clearly shows not only that Ancient Egypt and India were connected culturally but also spiritually. How does this knowledge help the spiritual aspirant? This discovery has great importance for the Yogis and mystics who follow the philosophy of Ancient Egypt and the mysticism of India. It means that India has a longer history and heritage than was previously understood. It shows that the mysteries of Ancient Egypt were essentially a yoga tradition which did not die but rather developed into the modern day systems of Yoga technology of India. It further shows that African culture developed Yoga Mysticism earlier than any other civilization in history. All of this expands our understanding of the unity of culture and the deep legacy of Yoga, which stretches into the distant past, beyond the Indus Valley civilization, the earliest known high culture in India as well as the Vedic tradition of Aryan culture. Therefore, Yoga culture and mysticism is the oldest known tradition of spiritual development and Indian mysticism is an extension of the Ancient Egyptian mysticism. By understanding the legacy which Ancient Egypt gave to India the mysticism of India is better understood and by comprehending the heritage of Indian Yoga, which is rooted in Ancient Egypt the Mysticism of Ancient Egypt is also better understood. This

The Ancient Egyptian Wisdom Texts

expanded understanding allows us to prove the underlying kinship of humanity, through the common symbols, motifs and philosophies which are not disparate and confusing teachings but in reality expressions of the same study of truth through metaphysics and mystical realization of Self. (HARD COVER) ISBN: 1-884564-50-X $45.00 U.S.   81/2" X 11"

6. AFRICAN ORIGINS BOOK 1 PART 1 African Origins of African Civilization, Religion, Yoga Mysticism and Ethics Philosophy-<u>Soft Cover</u> $24.95 ISBN: 1-884564-55-0

7. AFRICAN ORIGINS BOOK 2 PART 2 African Origins of Western Civilization, Religion and Philosophy (Soft) -<u>Soft Cover</u> $24.95 ISBN: 1-884564-56-9

8. EGYPT AND INDIA AFRICAN ORIGINS OF Eastern Civilization, Religion, Yoga Mysticism and Philosophy-<u>Soft Cover</u> $29.95 (Soft) ISBN: 1-884564-57-7

9. THE MYSTERIES OF ISIS: **The Ancient Egyptian Philosophy of Self-Realization** - There are several paths to discover the Divine and the mysteries of the higher Self. This volume details the mystery teachings of the goddess Aset (Isis) from Ancient Egypt- the path of wisdom. It includes the teachings of her temple and the disciplines that are enjoined for the initiates of the temple of Aset as they were given in ancient times. Also, this book includes the teachings of the main myths of Aset that lead a human being to spiritual enlightenment and immortality. Through the study of ancient myth and the illumination of initiatic understanding the idea of God is expanded from the mythological comprehension to the metaphysical. Then this metaphysical understanding is related to you, the student, so as to begin understanding your true divine nature. ISBN 1-884564-24-0 $22.99

10. EGYPTIAN PROVERBS: collection of —Ancient Egyptian Proverbs and Wisdom Teachings -How to live according to MAAT Philosophy. Beginning Meditation. All proverbs are indexed for easy searches. For the first time in one volume, ——Ancient Egyptian Proverbs, wisdom teachings and meditations, fully illustrated with hieroglyphic text and symbols. EGYPTIAN PROVERBS is a unique collection of knowledge and wisdom which you can put into practice today and transform your life. $14.95 U.S   ISBN: 1-884564-00-3

11. GOD OF LOVE: THE PATH OF DIVINE LOVE The Process of Mystical Transformation and The Path of Divine Love   This Volume focuses on the ancient wisdom teachings of "Neter Merri" –the Ancient Egyptian philosophy of Divine Love and how to use them in a scientific process for self-transformation.

The Ancient Egyptian Wisdom Texts

Love is one of the most powerful human emotions. It is also the source of Divine feeling that unifies God and the individual human being. When love is fragmented and diminished by egoism the Divine connection is lost. The Ancient tradition of Neter Merri leads human beings back to their Divine connection, allowing them to discover their innate glorious self that is actually Divine and immortal. This volume will detail the process of transformation from ordinary consciousness to cosmic consciousness through the integrated practice of the teachings and the path of Devotional Love toward the Divine. 5.5"x 8.5" ISBN 1-884564-11-9 $22.95

12. INTRODUCTION TO MAAT PHILOSOPHY: Spiritual Enlightenment Through the Path of Virtue   Known as Karma Yoga in India, the teachings of MAAT for living virtuously and with orderly wisdom are explained and the student is to begin practicing the precepts of Maat in daily life so as to promote the process of purification of the heart in preparation for the judgment of the soul. This judgment will be understood not as an event that will occur at the time of death but as an event that occurs continuously, at every moment in the life of the individual. The student will learn how to become allied with the forces of the Higher Self and to thereby begin cleansing the mind (heart) of impurities so as to attain a higher vision of reality. ISBN 1-884564-20-8 $22.99

13. MEDITATION The Ancient Egyptian Path to Enlightenment   Many people do not know about the rich history of meditation practice in Ancient Egypt. This volume outlines the theory of meditation and presents the Ancient Egyptian Hieroglyphic text which give instruction as to the nature of the mind and its three modes of expression. It also presents the texts which give instruction on the practice of meditation for spiritual Enlightenment and unity with the Divine. This volume allows the reader to begin practicing meditation by explaining, in easy to understand terms, the simplest form of meditation and working up to the most advanced form which was practiced in ancient times and which is still practiced by yogis around the world in modern times. ISBN 1-884564-27-7 $22.99

14. THE GLORIOUS LIGHT MEDITATION TECHNIQUE OF ANCIENT EGYPT New for the year 2000. This volume is based on the earliest known instruction in history given for the practice of formal meditation. Discovered by Dr. Muata Ashby, it is inscribed on the walls of the Tomb of Seti I in Thebes Egypt. This volume details the philosophy and practice of this unique system of meditation originated in Ancient Egypt and the earliest practice of meditation known in the world which occurred in the most advanced African Culture. ISBN: 1-884564-15-1 $16.95 (PB)

15. THE SERPENT POWER: The Ancient Egyptian Mystical Wisdom of the Inner Life Force.   This Volume specifically deals with the latent life Force energy of the universe and in the human body, its control and sublimation. How to

The Ancient Egyptian Wisdom Texts

develop the Life Force energy of the subtle body. This Volume will introduce the esoteric wisdom of the science of how virtuous living acts in a subtle and mysterious way to cleanse the latent psychic energy conduits and vortices of the spiritual body. ISBN 1-884564-19-4 $22.95

16. EGYPTIAN YOGA *The Postures of The Gods and Goddesses* Discover the physical postures and exercises practiced thousands of years ago in Ancient Egypt which are today known as Yoga exercises. Discover the history of the postures and how they were transferred from Ancient Egypt in Africa to India through Buddhist Tantrism. Then practice the postures as you discover the mythic teaching that originally gave birth to the postures and was practiced by the Ancient Egyptian priests and priestesses. This work is based on the pictures and teachings from the Creation story of Ra, The Asarian Resurrection Myth and the carvings and reliefs from various Temples in Ancient Egypt 8.5" X 11" ISBN 1-884564-10-0 Soft Cover $21.95   Exercise video $20

17. SACRED SEXUALITY: EGYPTIAN TANTRA YOGA: The Art of Sex Sublimation and Universal Consciousness This Volume will expand on the male and female principles within the human body and in the universe and further detail the sublimation of sexual energy into spiritual energy. The student will study the deities Min and Hathor, Asar and Aset, Geb and Nut and discover the mystical implications for a practical spiritual discipline. This Volume will also focus on the Tantric aspects of Ancient Egyptian and Indian mysticism, the purpose of sex and the mystical teachings of sexual sublimation which lead to self-knowledge and Enlightenment.   5.5"x 8.5"   ISBN 1-884564-03-8 $24.95

18. AFRICAN RELIGION Volume 4: ASARIAN THEOLOGY: RESURRECTING OSIRIS The path of Mystical Awakening and the Keys to Immortality NEW REVISED AND EXPANDED EDITION!   The Ancient Sages created stories based on human and superhuman beings whose struggles, aspirations, needs and desires ultimately lead them to discover their true Self. The myth of Aset, Asar and Heru is no exception in this area. While there is no one source where the entire story may be found, pieces of it are inscribed in various ancient Temples walls, tombs, steles and papyri. For the first time available, the complete myth of Asar, Aset and Heru has been compiled from original Ancient Egyptian, Greek and Coptic Texts. This epic myth has been richly illustrated with reliefs from the Temple of Heru at Edfu, the Temple of Aset at Philae, the Temple of Asar at Abydos, the Temple of Hathor at Denderah and various papyri, inscriptions and reliefs. Discover the myth which inspired the teachings of the *Shetaut Neter* (Egyptian Mystery System - Egyptian Yoga) and the Egyptian Book of Coming Forth By Day. Also, discover the three levels of Ancient Egyptian Religion, how to understand the mysteries of the Duat or Astral World and how to discover the abode of the Supreme in the Amenta, *The Other World* The ancient religion of Asar, Aset and Heru, if properly understood, contains all

The Ancient Egyptian Wisdom Texts

of the elements necessary to lead the sincere aspirant to attain immortality through inner self-discovery. This volume presents the entire myth and explores the main mystical themes and rituals associated with the myth for understating human existence, creation and the way to achieve spiritual emancipation - *Resurrection*. The Asarian myth is so powerful that it influenced and is still having an effect on the major world religions. Discover the origins and mystical meaning of the Christian Trinity, the Eucharist ritual and the ancient origin of the birthday of Jesus Christ. Soft Cover ISBN: 1-884564-27-5 $24.95

19. THE EGYPTIAN BOOK OF THE DEAD MYSTICISM OF THE PERT EM HERU " I Know myself, I know myself, I am One With God!–From the Pert Em Heru "The Ru Pert em Heru" or "Ancient Egyptian Book of The Dead," or "Book of Coming Forth By Day" as it is more popularly known, has fascinated the world since the successful translation of Ancient Egyptian hieroglyphic scripture over 150 years ago. The astonishing writings in it reveal that the Ancient Egyptians believed in life after death and in an ultimate destiny to discover the Divine. The elegance and aesthetic beauty of the hieroglyphic text itself has inspired many see it as an art form in and of itself. But is there more to it than that? Did the Ancient Egyptian wisdom contain more than just aphorisms and hopes of eternal life beyond death? In this volume Dr. Muata Ashby, the author of over 25 books on Ancient Egyptian Yoga Philosophy has produced a new translation of the original texts which uncovers a mystical teaching underlying the sayings and rituals instituted by the Ancient Egyptian Sages and Saints. "Once the philosophy of Ancient Egypt is understood as a mystical tradition instead of as a religion or primitive mythology, it reveals its secrets which if practiced today will lead anyone to discover the glory of spiritual self-discovery. The Pert em Heru is in every way comparable to the Indian Upanishads or the Tibetan Book of the Dead $28.95." ISBN# 1-884564-28-3 Size: 8½" X 11

20. African Religion VOL. 1- ANUNIAN THEOLOGY THE MYSTERIES OF RA The Philosophy of Anu and The Mystical Teachings of The Ancient Egyptian Creation Myth Discover the mystical teachings contained in the Creation Myth and the gods and goddesses who brought creation and human beings into existence. The Creation myth of Anu is the source of Anunian Theology but also of the other main theological systems of Ancient Egypt that also influenced other world religions including Christianity, Hinduism and Buddhism. The Creation Myth holds the key to understanding the universe and for attaining spiritual Enlightenment. ISBN: 1-884564-38-0 $19.95

21. African Religion VOL 3: Memphite Theology: MYSTERIES OF MIND Mystical Psychology & Mental Health for Enlightenment and Immortality based on the Ancient Egyptian Philosophy of Menefer -Mysticism of Ptah, Egyptian Physics and Yoga Metaphysics and the Hidden properties of Matter. This volume uncovers the mystical psychology of the

The Ancient Egyptian Wisdom Texts

Ancient Egyptian wisdom teachings centering on the philosophy of the Ancient Egyptian city of Menefer (Memphite Theology). How to understand the mind and how to control the senses and lead the mind to health, clarity and mystical self-discovery. This Volume will also go deeper into the philosophy of God as creation and will explore the concepts of modern science and how they correlate with ancient teachings. This Volume will lay the ground work for the understanding of the philosophy of universal consciousness and the initiatic/yogic insight into who or what is God? ISBN 1-884564-07-0 $22.95

22. AFRICAN RELIGION VOLUME 5: THE GODDESS AND THE EGYPTIAN MYSTERIESTHE PATH OF THE GODDESS THE GODDESS PATH The Secret Forms of the Goddess and the Rituals of Resurrection The Supreme Being may be worshipped as father or as mother. *Ushet Rekhat* or *Mother Worship*, is the spiritual process of worshipping the Divine in the form of the Divine Goddess. It celebrates the most important forms of the Goddess including *Nathor, Maat, Aset, Arat, Amentet and Hathor* and explores their mystical meaning as well as the rising of *Sirius,* the star of Aset (Aset) and the new birth of Hor (Heru). The end of the year is a time of reckoning, reflection and engendering a new or renewed positive movement toward attaining spiritual Enlightenment. The Mother Worship devotional meditation ritual, performed on five days during the month of December and on New Year's Eve, is based on the Ushet Rekhit. During the ceremony, the cosmic forces, symbolized by Sirius - and the constellation of Orion ---, are harnessed through the understanding and devotional attitude of the participant. This propitiation draws the light of wisdom and health to all those who share in the ritual, leading to prosperity and wisdom. $14.95 ISBN 1-884564-18-6

23. *THE MYSTICAL JOURNEY FROM JESUS TO CHRIST* Discover the ancient Egyptian origins of Christianity before the Catholic Church and learn the mystical teachings given by Jesus to assist all humanity in becoming Christlike. Discover the secret meaning of the Gospels that were discovered in Egypt. Also discover how and why so many Christian churches came into being. Discover that the Bible still holds the keys to mystical realization even though its original writings were changed by the church. Discover how to practice the original teachings of Christianity which leads to the Kingdom of Heaven. $24.95 ISBN# 1-884564-05-4 size: 8½" X 11"

24. THE STORY OF ASAR, ASET AND HERU: An Ancient Egyptian Legend (For Children)   Now for the first time, the most ancient myth of Ancient Egypt comes alive for children. Inspired by the books *The Asarian Resurrection: The Ancient Egyptian Bible* and *The Mystical Teachings of The Asarian Resurrection, The Story of Asar, Aset and Heru* is an easy to understand and thrilling tale which inspired the children of Ancient Egypt to aspire to greatness and righteousness.   If you and your child have enjoyed stories like *The Lion King* and *Star Wars you will love The Story of Asar, Aset and Heru.* Also, if you

The Ancient Egyptian Wisdom Texts

know the story of Jesus and Krishna you will discover than Ancient Egypt had a similar myth and that this myth carries important spiritual teachings for living a fruitful and fulfilling life. This book may be used along with *The Parents Guide To The Asarian Resurrection Myth: How to Teach Yourself and Your Child the Principles of Universal Mystical Religion*. The guide provides some background to the Asarian Resurrection myth and it also gives insight into the mystical teachings contained in it which you may introduce to your child. It is designed for parents who wish to grow spiritually with their children and it serves as an introduction for those who would like to study the Asarian Resurrection Myth in depth and to practice its teachings. 8.5" X 11"   ISBN: 1-884564-31-3 $12.95

25. THE PARENTS GUIDE TO THE AUSARIAN RESURRECTION MYTH: How to Teach Yourself and Your Child the Principles of Universal Mystical Religion. This insightful manual brings for the timeless wisdom of the ancient through the Ancient Egyptian myth of Asar, Aset and Heru and the mystical teachings contained in it for parents who want to guide their children to understand and practice the teachings of mystical spirituality. This manual may be used with the children's storybook *The Story of Asar, Aset and Heru* by Dr. Muata Abhaya Ashby.   ISBN: 1-884564-30-5 $16.95

26. HEALING THE CRIMINAL HEART. Introduction to Maat Philosophy, Yoga and Spiritual Redemption Through the Path of Virtue   Who is a criminal? Is there such a thing as a criminal heart? What is the source of evil and sinfulness and is there any way to rise above it? Is there redemption for those who have committed sins, even the worst crimes?   Ancient Egyptian mystical psychology holds important answers to these questions. Over ten thousand years ago mystical psychologists, the Sages of Ancient Egypt, studied and charted the human mind and spirit and laid out a path which will lead to spiritual redemption, prosperity and Enlightenment.   This introductory volume brings forth the teachings of the Asarian Resurrection, the most important myth of Ancient Egypt, with relation to the faults of human existence: anger, hatred, greed, lust, animosity, discontent, ignorance, egoism jealousy, bitterness, and a myriad of psycho-spiritual ailments which keep a human being in a state of negativity and adversity   ISBN: 1-884564-17-8 $15.95

27. TEMPLE RITUAL OF THE ANCIENT EGYPTIAN MYSTERIES-- THEATER & DRAMA OF THE ANCIENT EGYPTIAN MYSTERIES: Details the practice of the mysteries and ritual program of the temple and the philosophy an practice of the ritual of the mysteries, its purpose and execution. Featuring the Ancient Egyptian stage play-"The Enlightenment of Hathor' Based on an Ancient Egyptian Drama, The original Theater -Mysticism of the Temple of Hetheru 1-884564-14-3 $19.95   By Dr. Muata Ashby

The Ancient Egyptian Wisdom Texts

28. GUIDE TO PRINT ON DEMAND: SELF-PUBLISH FOR PROFIT, SPIRITUAL FULFILLMENT AND SERVICE TO HUMANITY Everyone asks us how we produced so many books in such a short time. Here are the secrets to writing and producing books that uplift humanity and how to get them printed for a fraction of the regular cost. Anyone can become an author even if they have limited funds. All that is necessary is the willingness to learn how the printing and book business work and the desire to follow the special instructions given here for preparing your manuscript format. Then you take your work directly to the non-traditional companies who can produce your books for less than the traditional book printer can. ISBN: 1-884564-40-2 $16.95 U. S.

29. Egyptian Mysteries: Vol. 1, Shetaut Neter What are the Mysteries? For thousands of years the spiritual tradition of Ancient Egypt, S*hetaut Neter,* "The Egyptian Mysteries," "The Secret Teachings," have fascinated, tantalized and amazed the world. At one time exalted and recognized as the highest culture of the world, by Africans, Europeans, Asiatics, Hindus, Buddhists and other cultures of the ancient world, in time it was shunned by the emerging orthodox world religions. Its temples desecrated, its philosophy maligned, its tradition spurned, its philosophy dormant in the mystical *Medu Neter*, the mysterious hieroglyphic texts which hold the secret symbolic meaning that has scarcely been discerned up to now. What are the secrets of *Nehast* {spiritual awakening and emancipation, resurrection}. More than just a literal translation, this volume is for awakening to the secret code *Shetitu* of the teaching which was not deciphered by Egyptologists, nor could be understood by ordinary spiritualists. This book is a reinstatement of the original science made available for our times, to the reincarnated followers of Ancient Egyptian culture and the prospect of spiritual freedom to break the bonds of *Khemn*, "ignorance," and slavery to evil forces: *Såaa* . ISBN: 1-884564-41-0 $19.99

30. EGYPTIAN MYSTERIES VOL 2: Dictionary of Gods and Goddesses This book is about the mystery of neteru, the gods and goddesses of Ancient Egypt (Kamit, Kemet). Neteru means "Gods and Goddesses." But the Neterian teaching of Neteru represents more than the usual limited modern day concept of "divinities" or "spirits." The Neteru of Kamit are also metaphors, cosmic principles and vehicles for the enlightening teachings of Shetaut Neter (Ancient Egyptian-African Religion). Actually they are the elements for one of the most advanced systems of spirituality ever conceived in human history. Understanding the concept of neteru provides a firm basis for spiritual evolution and the pathway for viable culture, peace on earth and a healthy human society. Why is it important to have gods and goddesses in our lives? In order for spiritual evolution to be possible, once a human being has accepted that there is existence after death and there is a transcendental being who exists beyond time and space knowledge, human beings need a connection to that which transcends the ordinary experience of human life in time and space and a means to

The Ancient Egyptian Wisdom Texts

understand the transcendental reality beyond the mundane reality. ISBN: 1-884564-23-2 $21.95

31. EGYPTIAN MYSTERIES VOL. 3 The Priests and Priestesses of Ancient Egypt This volume details the path of Neterian priesthood, the joys, challenges and rewards of advanced Neterian life, the teachings that allowed the priests and priestesses to manage the most long lived civilization in human history and how that path can be adopted today; for those who want to tread the path of the Clergy of Shetaut Neter. ISBN: 1-884564-53-4 $24.95

32. The War of Heru and Set: The Struggle of Good and Evil for Control of the World and The Human Soul This volume contains a novelized version of the Asarian Resurrection myth that is based on the actual scriptures presented in the Book Asarian Religion (old name –Resurrecting Osiris). This volume is prepared in the form of a screenplay and can be easily adapted to be used as a stage play. Spiritual seeking is a mythic journey that has many emotional highs and lows, ecstasies and depressions, victories and frustrations. This is the War of Life that is played out in the myth as the struggle of Heru and Set and those are mythic characters that represent the human Higher and Lower self. How to understand the war and emerge victorious in the journey o life? The ultimate victory and fulfillment can be experienced, which is not changeable or lost in time. The purpose of myth is to convey the wisdom of life through the story of divinities who show the way to overcome the challenges and foibles of life. In this volume the feelings and emotions of the characters of the myth have been highlighted to show the deeply rich texture of the Ancient Egyptian myth. This myth contains deep spiritual teachings and insights into the nature of self, of God and the mysteries of life and the means to discover the true meaning of life and thereby achieve the true purpose of life. To become victorious in the battle of life means to become the King (or Queen) of Egypt.Have you seen movies like The Lion King, Hamlet, The Odyssey, or The Little Buddha? These have been some of the most popular movies in modern times. The Sema Institute of Yoga is dedicated to researching and presenting the wisdom and culture of ancient Africa. The Script is

The Ancient Egyptian Wisdom Texts

designed to be produced as a motion picture but may be addapted for the theater as well. $21.95 copyright 1998 By Dr. Muata Ashby ISBN 1-8840564-44-5

33. AFRICAN DIONYSUS: FROM EGYPT TO GREECE: The Kamitan Origins of Greek Culture and Religion ISBN: 1-884564-47-X FROM EGYPT TO GREECE This insightful manual is a reference to Ancient Egyptian mythology and philosophy and its correlation to what later became known as Greek and Rome mythology and philosophy. It outlines the basic tenets of the mythologies and shoes the ancient origins of Greek culture in Ancient Egypt. This volume also documents the origins of the Greek alphabet in Egypt as well as Greek religion, myth and philosophy of the gods and goddesses from Egypt from the myth of Atlantis and archaic period with the Minoans to the Classical period. This volume also acts as a resource for Colleges students who would like to set up fraternities and sororities based on the original Ancient Egyptian principles of Sheti and Maat philosophy. ISBN: 1-884564-47-X $22.95 U.S.

34. THE FORTY TWO PRECEPTS OF MAAT, THE PHILOSOPHY OF RIGHTEOUS ACTION AND THE ANCIENT EGYPTIAN WISDOM TEXTS <u>ADVANCED STUDIES</u> This manual is designed for use with the 1998 Maat Philosophy Class conducted by Dr. Muata Ashby. This is a detailed study of Maat Philosophy. It contains a compilation of the 42 laws or precepts of Maat and the corresponding principles which they represent along with the teachings of the ancient Egyptian Sages relating to each. Maat philosophy was the basis of Ancient Egyptian society and government as well as the heart of Ancient Egyptian myth and spirituality. Maat is at once a goddess, a cosmic force and a living social doctrine, which promotes social harmony and thereby paves the way for spiritual evolution in all levels of society. ISBN: 1-884564-48-8 $16.95 U.S.

35. **THE SECRET LOTUS:** *Poetry of Enlightenment*

The Ancient Egyptian Wisdom Texts

Discover the mystical sentiment of the Kemetic teaching as expressed through the poetry of Sebai Muata Ashby. The teaching of spiritual awakening is uniquely experienced when the poetic sensibility is present. This first volume contains the poems written between 1996 and 2003. **1-884564--16 -X $16.99**

The Ancient Egyptian Wisdom Texts

Order Form

Telephone orders: Call Toll Free: 1(305) 378-6253. Have your AMEX, Optima, Visa or MasterCard ready.
    Fax orders: 1-(305) 378-6253   E-MAIL ADDRESS: Semayoga@aol.com
Postal Orders: Sema Institute of Yoga, P.O. Box 570459, Miami, Fl. 33257. USA.
    Please send the following books and / or tapes.

ITEM
_____Cost $_____
_____Cost $_____
_____Cost $_____
_____Cost $_____
_____Cost $_____
                                          Total $_____
Name:_____

Physical Address:_____

City:_____ State:_____ Zip:_____

Sales tax: Please add 6.5% for books shipped to Florida addresses
_____Shipping: $6.50 for first book and .50¢ for each additional
_____Shipping: Outside US $5.00 for first book and $3.00 for each additional

_____Payment:_____
_____Check -Include Driver License #:
      _____

_____Credit card: _____ Visa, _____ MasterCard, _____ Optima, _____ AMEX.

Card number:_____
Name on card:_____ Exp. date:_____/_____

Copyright 1995-2005 Dr. R. Muata Abhaya Ashby
Sema Institute of Yoga
P.O.Box 570459, Miami, Florida, 33257
(305) 378-6253 Fax: (305) 378-6253

www.ingramcontent.com/pod-product-compliance
Lightning Source LLC
Chambersburg PA
CBHW021108080526
44587CB00010B/434